YOU SAY GOODBYE AND WE SAY HELLO:

The Montessori Method for Positive Dementia Care

Tom and Karen Brenner

Table of Contents

DEDICATION

This book is dedicated to the many people who helped us make this dream come true:

OUR FAMILY:

Frankie, who designed our beautiful book cover and art work.

Julia, who spent hours editing our book as well as being our photographer.

Chad, who formatted our book layout and created our web site.

Gwen and Kathryn who materially and emotionally supported us.

Henri and Yuki who sat patiently by us at the computer hour after hour.

OUR FRIENDS:

Diane, road warrior who traveled through rain, wind and snow with us.

Jean, who believed in us first.

All of the wonderful people at:

Peabody Retirement Community, The Danish Home, Rush Alzheimer's Family Care Center, Family Alliance, Swan Creek Retirement Community, The Birches Assisted Living, The Greater Chicago Alzheimer's Association, The Juliana Group, Seton Montessori Institute, The American Montessori Society, The Frank and Laura Smock Foundation, Bob DeMarco (and Dotty), *Editor and Founder, Alzheimer's Reading Room*, Betsey Odell, *Vice President, Fisher Center for Alzheimer's Research Foundation*

We are so very grateful to all of you! We are blessed to have you in our lives.

Tom & Karen Brenner
Chicago, 2012

ACKNOWLEDGMENT

We have been fortunate to work in long term care homes, adult day centers and memory clinics in cities, farm communities and suburbs. In these various settings, we have worked with people from all walks of life, different races, ethnicities, religions and philosophies. We believe that people facing many different situations will find guidance and inspiration in the stories featured in our book. While the people we write about are real people, we have changed their names and their situations to protect their privacy and the privacy of their caregivers and families. To all of the people who worked with us (both people living with dementia and their caregivers) we are truly and humbly grateful. Without your help and support, we could not have written this book.

We also want to acknowledge here our use of the Beatles' song titles throughout our book. The Beatles were the soundtrack to our lives when we were coming of age. Now that we are the generation that is caring for others and/or being cared for by others, the Beatles' music once again helps us tell our stories.

–Tom & Karen

INTRODUCTION:

The Long and Winding Road

Bill's Story:

I wish there was someone I could talk to about this. Everyone here is very nice to us, they take good care of Bill, but they don't really know him; I mean they don't know the real man inside. What can I do? No one wants to hear the stories about Bill, about how he was a high school football star and a hero in the war. I just wish there was some way I could tell the people here, I wish I could show them what a strong, brave man Bill is.

I still remember the feeling of shock when he asked me to wear his letterman jacket our senior year, how that jacket felt in my hands, how it smelled of leather and wool. It was dark blue wool with white leather sleeves. Bill's name and number were embroidered on the back, right under the roaring lion. I used to sleep with that jacket every night my senior year in high school. Even though he was the star quarterback, Bill was still shy. He told me later that he was self conscious because his ears stuck out and turned red when he got embarrassed. I didn't care about football, I was a book worm.

It was Bill's smile that got me, he just kind of lights up when he grins. I used to love it, too, when he would pass me in the hall and give me that grin and then a wink, made my heart beat fast!

I didn't know what to feel when Bill joined the Marines right after high school. We were just getting serious and he was going to leave me. I felt angry and sad and proud all at the same time. Everyone was joining up or getting drafted then. Of course in those days, we didn't question anything; we just did what we were told. I could not believe it when his mother called me to tell me that Billy had run into a little trouble over there. A little trouble? He almost died saving the company medic, Henry Brooks. Henry was hit bad and Bill picked him up out of a fox hole and ran through the middle of a battle and carried him to safety. Henry went on to become a doctor, and to save a lot of lives himself. Now, Dr. Henry is dead and no one remembers what my Bill did, how he saved that doctor's life, how he won medals for his bravery. Bill told me later it was all that running, dodging and weaving that he did on the football field that saved them both. He didn't think it was bravery. Bill just chalked it up to speed and luck.

And the Lord knows Bill was quick on his feet and in his mind. They used to call him jackrabbit. People said he was so fast, he could throw the football and then catch his own pass! Even though he was quick in everything, Bill had patience for other people. He helped a lot of kids, boys that would have gone bad if it wasn't for Bill. They come sometimes to visit us here, but they look so sad when they see how Bill is now. Of course, it's hard for our own kids to visit, too. They don't know how to handle seeing their dad like this. I know it's hard for them, but they have to understand that their father is still there, inside. I don't know what to say to them, to help them understand this. I don't know what to say to anybody.

I know that people sometimes think I am mean because I won't help Bill button his shirt and I won't let anyone feed him. It's just that I know Bill, and I know that he feels better about himself when he can do these things on his own. I am trying to be as patient with Bill as he always was with other people. I know that he will never get any better, but I want him to put up a fight. I want us to put up a fight for as long as we can.

Now Bill is beginning to wake up from his nap. He needs to sit up straighter in his wheel chair, and he needs to wipe his chin. Oh, he sees me now. There is that old grin and Lord, feel my heart, he winked at me! My Bill, my hero.

- The End

This story is apocryphal; it is the voice of a woman who represents many caregivers. This central theme, that of a woman who still sees her husband as the heroic man she fell in love with, is a story that we hear over and over in our work. We have been working together in the dementia field for many years and have found a variety of true stories of heroes who are now living with dementia. These stories deeply touch our own lives.

The stories we hear in our work with elders demonstrate that people who have dementia still possess the wisdom and the spirit that helped them create such rich lives. It is often difficult to access these stories, but just because it is not always easy to reach people with dementia, it does not mean that the effort isn't worth it. As long as we live, we all have a need to tell our stories.

You Say Goodbye and We Say Hello includes stories from the lives of poets, pastors, farmers, teachers, scientists, and musicians: all of them are living with dementia. We have worked with people who have traveled the world and people who never left the family farm. For each person, the dementia journey is different. We have found people who are willing to share some of their life's gifts with us, even with all of the difficulties, the frustrations and the fear that often accompanies dementia. We are now and forever grateful to these wonderful, brave, and giving people. Their stories remind us that dementia defines a set of symptoms, but it does not define a life.

Dementia is not something that we would wish on the people we love, or on ourselves, but it does not have to be the terrible fate that is often described in books, articles, and movies. We have become used to thinking in purely negative terms when it comes to dementia. It may be surprising, but it is true that there is a more positive approach to be found in caring for people who have dementia. We cannot change the diagnosis, we cannot cure the symptoms of dementia, but we can change our expectations. We can learn to be in the moment, to follow the rhythm and the patterns of people living with dementia. This is not familiar territory, but it is not impossible terrain. There is a path that we can follow through the journey of dementia. This book will help you find your own path. The first step on this journey is to rethink the negative and doom laden language that is often used to describe dementia.

People with dementia are not the walking dead, being in a relationship with someone who happens to have this condition is not just one long good bye. We have to find a new way to say hello; it is our job to find a way to be in relationship. It is our gift to help people with dementia stay connected to those who love and care for them.

One of the most dynamic and effective tools we have for helping people with dementia stay connected is by listening to, collecting, and sharing their stories. Moments when patients are sharing their stories are moments when they are present with us. These moments, no matter how brief or how fleeting, can be times of great meaning and wonderful, deeply felt connection. We understand that people who are living with dementia struggle with declining physical abilities as well as loss of memory and cognitive decline, but we have also found that while the mind and body may grow weaker, the spirit can, and often does, grow stronger. It is these moments of soul-to-soul connection that are captured in the stories that people tell us. It is through these stories that the spirit of the people we meet in our work comes shining through the fog of dementia.

Over the years of working with people who are living with dementia, we have developed a memory support program that has been very successful in reaching people who may seem unreachable. We will demonstrate in this book how you can replicate our method at home or when you visit your loved one in an intentional community. Our goal is to help you stay connected with the person you love, to honor their lives by acknowledging the person who still lives inside of them.

In our book, *You Say Good Bye and We Say Hello,* we not only share the stories of people living with dementia, we share with you the techniques and tools that we have developed to help you stay connected to the people you love. We have researched and field tested our memory support program in long-term care homes, adult day centers, memory enhancement centers, and private homes for over ten years. Our program, The Montessori Method for Positive Dementia Care, can be successfully used by family caregivers, medical staff, front line care staff, and therapists.

It is a program designed to be accessible and cost effective. The Montessori Method for Positive Dementia

Care provides support for elders with dementia and is also very supportive of their caregivers.

Reading this book will provide you with a better understanding of dementia as well as giving you the tools and ideas you need for staying connected to the person you care for. Our book will be supportive of you, whether you are a family caregiver or a professional care person. We will help you face the challenges of caregiving and help you find those fleeting moments of connection.

We have traveled down the dementia road with many, many people. These journeys have shown us the twists and turns, valleys and peaks of this long and winding road. We will share with you the important guideposts we have discovered on this road. Here is a story of our very first journey into the world of dementia:

Tom and Karen's Story:

The couple, a man and woman, stood just outside the door of the Scandinavian Home, arguing. The autumn leaves from the towering elms on the grounds of the nursing home swirled around their feet as the cold wind snatched their voices away.

"I told you Tom, I don't want to go back today. I am afraid of some of those people. You know how much I hate scenes and last Saturday Bridget yelled at us and told us that nobody wanted us there. I just froze when she took off her slipper and

started hitting that other woman on the head with it. You knew what to do, how to calm her down, I just stood there, completely frozen. Anyway, I don't know what I'm doing, I'm just a Montessori teacher, you're the gerontologist, you're the specialist on aging, you're the one who spent the last six years researching dementia. I'm not going in. I'll wait in the car for you."

He took her hand.

"I know this is kind of scary sometimes, but what about the other thing that happened last Saturday? You know, when you had everyone singing together, even Don, who never says a word. He was singing and clapping and for a few minutes, he was connected again. That's why we're here, that's what we do."

"I know, Tom, I know that's what we're supposed to do, to help people reconnect, but I am so much more comfortable in a room full of little kids. You're the expert, not me. I don't know what I'm dong."

"Come on, Karen, we're in this thing together. We'll learn how to do this as we go. We're a great team, aren't we? I mean, we've been married forever, we've raised great kids, so we can do this together, too."

"Right, a great team. If we're so great at this, how come Bridget hates us? Anyway, we argue all the time, we're arguing now. What makes you think we can work together?"

He picked up her hand again.

"Because we are meant to do this, because we beat cancer together, because I can't do this without you."

He pushed open the door and pulled her in with him and with his lopsided smile whispered to her, "Anyway, Bridget doesn't hate us, Bridget hates you!"

When they walked in the door of the Scandinavian Home that Saturday afternoon, Bridget was once again hitting Elsa over the head with her slipper. Bridget's bright orange hair stood up around her head as though the anger in her body was electrifying her hair. Elsa, much smaller and older than Bridget stood meekly, her only movement a slight raising of her shoulders as Bridget's slipper rained blows on her head. Karen stood rooted to the ground, she was afraid of Bridget on her good days; she had no idea what to do with Bridget when she was violent. There was no staff around, no other visitors, just Tom and Karen. Tom walked calmly up to Bridget and put his hand on her raised arm.

"Every thing is OK, Bridget. You can stop now."

"You aren't my doctor, are you?" She asked and looked up at Tom through narrowed eyes.

"No, but I am your friend, and everything is fine now."
Bridget jerked her arm out of Tom's grip and straightened her posture with an attempt to regain some semblance of dignity. She sat heavily on a nearby chair and put her slipper back on

her foot and then stomped away without any apology to Elsa or any acknowledgement of Tom and Karen. Elsa rubbed her head and tears began to fall down her wrinkled, papery cheeks. Tom led her to a comfortable seat and began to talk quietly to Elsa while Karen went in search of a nurse or an aide or someone who could help Elsa. Her knees were shaking. What on earth were they doing here?

That was the way we began our work in dementia care, learning from our mistakes, finding out what worked and trying to understand why it worked. We have had the enormous good fortune of meeting people with dementia who were kind and patient and generous with us. We also met lots of 'Bridgets', people who wanted nothing to do with us, who were difficult, sometimes violent. We learned from these hard cases that if we didn't give up on them, we could find a way to reach even them.

With Bridget, it was a simple video camera that did the trick. She recognized that it was a camera and that we were making a film. Suddenly, Bridget was full of charm as she sashayed back in forth in front of the camera, smiling and glancing coyly over her shoulder at the lens. That was the very important lesson that Bridget taught us: Be prepared to be surprised!

Through field testing the Montessori Method for dementia care, we found out what absolutely would not work and we discovered what worked really well. For us, success is measured in a smile, wide awake eyes, laughter; some sign, no matter how small, that we are helping people with dementia connect once again. We have learned to be careful observers, to see the tiny step forward, the small improvement, the flash of joy. We know that we cannot cure the condition or bring back a fully functioning person, but we can share with you our experiences of discovery and connection. The simple but often profound discoveries that we have made on this dementia journey are highlighted in the book by guideposts. These guideposts will help you find your way on your own journey, your own long and winding road.

Our book is designed to take each step along this road with you, to help you regain your footing when you falter, to encourage you to celebrate each tiny victory, to remind you that caregiving is a calling of the highest order. You are giving the person you care for the greatest gift of all: your time, your love, your best effort.

CHAPTER ONE:

The Magical Mystery Tour

SOMEONE YOU LOVE has just been diagnosed with dementia. You may feel that this is the end of life as you know it. You are probably awash in the ocean of negativity that is out there when people speak of dementia. There is the look of pain, of sympathy, the "there but for the grace of God" attitude that well-meaning friends and family feel they must convey to people living with dementia. You will be told over and over, and you will read over and over again, about the walking dead, the long good bye, the loneliness, the exhaustion, the fear, the dread, the…STOP! There are always choices in life. You still have a life and you can still make choices. Of course, there is no cure for dementia, but there is a path, a way for you through this dementia journey.

Having dementia does not have to mean that your life is over; it does mean your life will be different. We make our plans for our life: when we get to be *this* age, we will do *this*, when we have accomplished *this*, then we will be able to do *that*. Life has a funny way of changing and re-purposing our grand designs, our hopes and dreams. Dementia is not a condition that anyone wants to face or confront, but you have been dealt these cards and now you must find a way to live with dementia and continue living your life as fully as possible.

The magical mystery tour of dementia is all new territory, and it is different for each person. You will have to decide how you are going to take this journey, but you should know that you are never alone, no matter how wild the ride, how frightening the road. It is important to reach out to friends and loved ones and invite them to take this trip with you. You will have to be the one who reaches out. Oftentimes, when friends and family hear the words "Alzheimer's and dementia" they don't know how to react; they don't know what to say or what to do. People sometimes react to the news of dementia the same way they deal with death. They become mute, they feel awkward, they want to flee, and they sometimes act as though it is contagious! You will be the one who has to assure friends and family that the dementia journey is not about death, it is about life. You will have to tell people you trust and love that this is not the time to say good-bye, this is the time to say hello. Invite people just to show up, visit, talk, play cards, eat a meal, or go for a walk. This is not about the end; this is about a beginning.

It will be up to you to engage your friends and family, to tell them what you need and when you need it.

Your ego, your pride and even parts of your privacy will have to be thrown under the bus before you can begin this tour. This is understandably hard for many of us. We are all trained in this culture to be fiercely independent, to be strong and capable. Many of us believe that asking for help is a sign of weakness. We don't want to burden anyone. However, when you ask another person for help, or when you tell another person how you are truly feeling, you give them a great gift; you give them the opportunity to be compassionate, to come to the aid of another human being. In our increasingly isolated and busy lives, many people don't often have the opportunity to practice that most human quality, coming to the aid of another. When we ask for help, we also give someone else the chance to be in a state of grace, the grace of giving of one's time, or energy, or compassion.

> # GUIDEPOST:
> Asking for help provides others with the opportunity to be in a state of grace.

Over the years of working with people who are living with dementia, we have learned a few rules of the road.

We'll call these rules **guideposts.** Some of these guideposts will seem glaringly obvious, some may seem strange or obscure, but they are all tested by us, and we know how helpful these guideposts can be on the dementia journey.

GUIDEPOST:

Take one step at a time.

A good rule of thumb when preparing for the dementia journey is to remember that it doesn't help you or anyone else if you are trying to control what will happen tomorrow, or next month, or next year when you, in truth, cannot control what will happen the next moment. When facing dementia, you can't control what will happen, but you can prepare. Being prepared means seeking out all the information that you can find. This will help you better understand the journey that you are taking. Professional groups, such as the Alzheimer's Association, can be very helpful in giving you free, educational materials.

GUIDEPOST:

Educate yourself.

There are many support groups for those who are living with dementia and their loved ones and friends. There are also many informational and support groups available online. Some Internet dementia support groups that we recommend are *The Fisher Alzheimer's Research Center Website and blog*[1], *The Alzheimer's Reading Room*[2], and *Caregiving.com.* Many religious leaders and professional counselors are also trained in support for people living with dementia. Please do not be shy about talking about your fears, concerns, and questions with your friends and family. You cannot take this trip alone; get everyone you need on the bus with you.

GUIDEPOST:

Gather a support group.

Okay, so these guideposts (take one step at a time, educate yourself, gather a support group) are things that many people know about; this is not new information. It isn't new, but it is the beginning of a new conversation, a new way of looking at dementia and the people who are living with it. Do you notice that we keep saying *living with dementia*? This is deliberate.

---

[1] http://www.alzinfo.org/

[2] http://www.alzheimersreadingroom.com/

People living with dementia can still have a life, and so can their care givers.

We want to change the language that surrounds dementia and the way that you and those in your life talk about dementia. There is so much power in language. Our words frame the way we look at our lives and the way that others look at our lives. If we choose to talk about ourselves and our loved ones as victims, or as martyrs, then that that is how others will see us and how we will begin to see ourselves. Choosing martyrdom or victimhood isn't helpful to you or to anyone in your life. You can begin to see yourself and to see dementia in a whole new light by first changing the dialogue, the language in your life.

One of the first things you can do to help change the tapes that play in your head is to listen to yourself and how you discuss dementia. Do you tend to discuss the life you are leading now in negative terms? Do you find yourself saying or thinking, "Dementia is taking over my life." Or, "Dementia is destroying my life." You certainly have a right to those feelings, those words, but what good does it do you to dwell on negative feelings? Where do you go from there? How does negative thinking help you or your loved one? It doesn't.

What would happen if you changed the dialogue to something like, "Dementia has made my life very different"? This statement can lead to all sorts of possibilities, some good, and some bad. How is your life different living with dementia? Do you find that sometimes you feel closer to the people you love? Do you find that you are learning to live in the moment? To appreciate things you once took for granted? You might also feel that some very important parts of your life are now and forever lost. That is true, but there are parts of your life that are more precious than ever before; there are parts of your life now that are wacky and weird, strange and sometimes scary.

All of these emotions are understandable; you are on the magical mystery tour of dementia. This is a journey that is never the same for any two people. You have to figure out how you are going to make this trip. We are here to help you find your way. There is a path through dementia world. While we don't have all the answers, we do have guideposts to help you. We also have well-researched and positive techniques for you to use to help navigate this journey that you did not choose, but that you must complete.

The idea of a *magical* mystery tour may seem wrong-headed and insensitive to you as you struggle to make sense of this trip that you did not choose to take. The word magical may mean different things to different people. To us, it means that this dementia journey is completely unpredictable. Those touchstones that we count on for reassurance in relationships are turned on their heads in dementia world. The loving person we have known for years may disappear for a while and then, suddenly, pop up again in the most unexpected way, or when we least expect to see that aspect of them again. This sort of magic is often found in very brief, fleeting moments; moments of profound wisdom, or an unexpected, revelatory statement. We understand that these moments of magic, of the elusive glimpse of the person we love, do not necessarily bring tremendous comfort to us, but these magical moments of connection do remind us of why we are on this magical mystery dementia tour.

The mystery of dementia is, of course, very plain to anyone who is on the dementia trip. There is so much that is not understood about this condition by both medical professionals and family caregivers. We often think that we have a handle on the situation only to find in the next moment that everything has changed again. The only way to live with dementia is to live one moment at a time, trying to understand, appreciate and enjoy that moment. To try and see the long view, or to try and understand the whole of dementia is too much for most of us, the unknowns are too profound, the mystery is too great. We have to embrace each small step along this journey. We look only at the road in front of us, not the road behind us, nor the long, winding road off in the distance, just the small space directly in front of us. We have to keep putting one foot in front of the other, celebrating those small moments that come as a flash of joy or recognition, and keep believing that, though the dementia journey is a tough one, it is all worth it.

You will need to travel light, and learn how to be flexible, to find new routes to familiar places, to throw away all of the old maps, all of the old guides. You are on a trip that will demand all of your patience, your stamina, your love. There will be tremendous sadness and frustration and weariness on this journey, but there will also be amazing magic and wondrous mysteries and yes, even joy. It is not the journey you had planned, but it will be amazing. Your family, friends, support groups, doctors, and the two of us are taking this magical mystery tour with you. Buckle up!

CHAPTER TWO:

Got to Get You into My Life

IT IS OFTEN said of dementia that this condition robs people of their personhood, it takes away their memories and abilities, and so the reasoning goes that dementia destroys the person's life. We have met and worked with hundreds of people living with dementia and the families who love and care for them. There is so much pain and hurt that surrounds this dementia journey. Wives often feel that if their husband no longer appears to recognize them or remember their name, then it means he no longer loves them, that they have lost the love of their life. It is true, a spouse may not seem to know their loved one, a mother may seem not to remember her own children. Can we understand what is going on here? Can we put aside our own feelings of abandonment, hurt and anger and try to understand what is happening to the people we love? If someone cannot remember their own life, then who are they? Are they still our husband, our wife, our mother, father, friend? The question is, can a person still be who they are and not remember who they were?

Are we a series of events, or do we have unique qualities that make us who we are?

After years of doing this work, we have found that people living with dementia are still the people they always were. But, how can that be, when they don't seem to know their own families, when they don't remember their own children's names? Is remembering all we are? Is a person lost to us because they don't remember their wedding day, or the job they held for thirty years? Is there some other handle we can find to hold onto, to have a relationship with someone who doesn't seem to know us?

At this point in the dementia journey, we have to throw our egos under the bus. We have to be willing to meet the person we love exactly where they are in the dementia journey. If this means that they don't seem to know us, then we have the privilege of introducing ourselves to them and letting them get to know us again. This may seem a very lonely and heartbreaking act, to introduce ourselves to our mother or father or husband or wife as though we were strangers. It *is* lonely and heartbreaking! It is also compassionate, liberating and sometimes very funny. This re-introducing ourselves all the time gives us the opportunity to drop a lot of baggage that families tend to carry over the years. We get a new beginning every time we meet.

If we take the time to try and understand what is happening to the person we love, it will help us learn how to take this lack of recognition less personally. This may seem like a rather harsh or impossible statement, but we have seen that when family members begin to gather more knowledge about dementia and how it affects the mind, then with that understanding comes some measure of comfort. We will take a moment here and give you a brief, but hopefully helpful explanation of how dementia may affect the mind.

Did you know that there are different memory systems at work in our brains? In this section, we will focus on how two memory systems are impacted by dementia: the declarative memory system and the procedural memory system. We want to share this information with you so that you can better understand the course of the dementia journey. Having some understanding of why a person with dementia may not be able to remember names, or remember that they just ate dinner, may not make the feeling of being hurt or being frustrated go away, but having an understanding of what is happening can help alleviate some of the pain and frustration.

Part of the reason that a person with dementia may ask the same question over and over again is because the memory system that tends to be most affected by this condition is the declarative memory. This is the memory system that affects short term memory, language, facts, recent episodes and executive function. This is why a person living with dementia often cannot remember things that happened five minutes ago.

GUIDEPOST:

Forget the word 'remember.'

For someone living with dementia, it is as though someone walks in every five minutes with a magic wand, waves the wand, and poof, everything that just happened to them in the last few minutes disappears. This disappearing act happens every few minutes, all day long. Can you imagine how frustrating, how frightening, how aggravating this must be?

It is often made even worse by well-meaning caregivers who insist that the person:

"Just ate ten minutes ago, don't you remember?"

"Just saw your daughter this morning, don't you remember?"

"Just went outside for a walk, don't you remember?"

The problem is, of course, that people with dementia *don't* remember these episodes that just happened. That magic wand wipes the slate clean again, and again, and again.

To make our lives and the lives of people living with dementia a bit easier, we recommend that you lose the word "remember." This is not an easy thing to do. In the course of a conversation, it is very natural to ask each other if we remember a person or event. But, for the person living with Alzheimer's, asking them to remember is like asking them to jump up and fly around the room. It is an impossible request and we must be vigilant in avoiding direct requests for information recall. When people with dementia are asked to remember something, this request can make them anxious or frustrated and may cause them to become very angry, depressed or withdrawn.

> # GUIDEPOST:
>
> Declarative memory system affects short term memory, language, facts, recent episodes and executive function.

Declarative memory also affects language, and that is why people living with Dementia often struggle to remember names of people or names of common objects.

We all do a little of this ourselves in our daily lives. We've all had the experience where a word is right on the tip of our tongue but we cannot find it. Later, sometimes in the middle of the night, we'll bolt up in bed and shout, "Calculus! He was good at *calculus*," finally remembering that elusive word. This is very common, especially in our overloaded and frantic lives. But, for the person living with Alzheimer's, the constant struggle for words can be exhausting and enraging.

Many times when we are working in a nursing home or an adult day center, we will hear family members or friends pleading with their loved one who has dementia,

"You remember, Mom. They lived next door to us for forty years! You have to remember them. She was your best friend!"

Because of the impaired declarative memory, people with dementia are often not able to remember names or faces of people they have known most of their lives. Trying to convince them otherwise is not going to help. We have to understand what they are dealing with; there are parts of their memory that are simply gone.

As is often the case on the dementia journey, just when we think we have a handle on understanding, something wild and unexpected happens. We may have worked hard to forget the word "remember," when suddenly the person we love remembers us or some event from their lives. This may last only a few seconds, or a few minutes, but it is like the sunlight breaking through the clouds when it is happens. For a fleeting moment, we have the person we knew and loved with us again. Then, heartbreakingly, it is gone; the light goes out, the cloud descends.

GUIDEPOST:

Celebrate each moment of recognition, each gesture of connection, every laugh, and every smile.

To keep the ones we love in our life, it is important to understand that these fleeting moments of recognition or remembrance are causes for celebration, not despair. Rather than constantly mourning the loss of the person we knew and loved, we must learn to appreciate these brief encounters, these moments of connection. We must learn to see them as little gifts that flash brightly and leave just as suddenly as they come. If we can learn to enjoy this flash of connection, these little moments, we can have the people we love in our lives again, not, of course, as we used to have them in our lives, but still with us, one brief moment at a time. These moments of recognition, of connection, are like little jewels that are strung on the necklace of time.

Laverne's Story:

This flash of connection happened in a most unusual way one day when we were working with Laverne. We had known Laverne for over a year. She had never spoken more than a one or two word phrase in our presence. She would often break into song, or come out with some 1920's slang, "bee's knees" being one of her favorites. One day, as we were working with a group of people in the dementia locked unit where Laverne was living, one of the nurses told us that Laverne had been speaking some foreign language all day. They had called her brother on the telephone to ask if the family spoke another language, but Laverne's brother assured them that the family had only spoken only English, and as far as he knew, Laverne had never learned another language.

We went to sit with Laverne to see if we could understand what was going on with her. At first, Laverne seemed much as usual, she would speak the occasional short phrase, or sing snatches of an old Broadway song. Then, she turned to us and, looking directly at us, began to recite the prologue to Chaucer's Canterbury Tales! She started to falter when she reached the line,

OF WHICH VIRTUE ENGENDER'D IS THE FLOWER.

Laverne seemed to be stuck on the word "virtue."

Fortunately, we remembered some of the prologue and were able to help Laverne finish the line. She looked at us very steadily with her light blue eyes, smiled and nodded decisively,

"You got that right!" she told us by way of thanks.

We never heard Laverne speak more than her standard two or three words again and she never again recited Chaucer, but that one day, from the depths of her memory, she remembered an old high school assignment. Laverne's astonishing recitation did not change her circumstances but it helped us, and the staff caring for her, remember that she was once a young high school girl, sitting in English class learning about Chaucer and Middle English. These sorts of breakthroughs, these flashes of light, these brief moments of lucidity or recognition do not change anything, but they give us glimpses of the whole person. These moments are causes for celebration, not sadness! We can keep the person we love in our lives if we are willing to have them with us for five seconds, five minutes or for just one look, one gesture, one kiss.

GUIDEPOST:

A magic wand is waved every five minutes and all the events of the last few minutes vanish, poof!

As we mentioned before, the declarative memory system also affects recent episodes or events. This is why someone living with dementia may ask the same question over and over again. They may not remember that they just ate lunch, or that their grandchildren just came to visit. Asking questions over and over and forgetting something that just happened can be very frustrating for everyone, the person living with dementia and the people who love them. Demanding that someone remember that they just ate lunch, or getting irritated with them because they can't remember things that have just happened are counter-productive for all involved. We are going to provide you with useful, practical techniques to help you and the person living with dementia learn how to cope with failing short term memory. We have worked for many years in memory support and find that these techniques, while simple, can be very effective. Once you understand what is going on in the memory systems of a person living with dementia, you can begin to develop your own personal coping strategies and techniques for keeping the person you love in your life.

Dementia also tends to affect the part of the declarative memory system where we store facts and common knowledge. So, a person living with dementia may not remember general knowledge or common facts. They may have been a person who was very involved in politics and now cannot tell you the name of the president of the United States. They may have worked as a carpenter and now cannot remember how many inches are in a foot. This does not mean that dementia robs someone of their intellect. This lack of general knowledge and facts does not mean that the person living with dementia is now suddenly stupid; it means that the person living with dementia still has possession of this knowledge; it is just much more difficult or impossible for them to access this knowledge.

We have worked with people who understood that they had lost the ability to access knowledge that once informed their lives on a daily basis. They would tell us that they felt stupid or slow, or that their heads weren't working right anymore. When a person realizes that they have difficulty in accessing knowledge that used to be at their fingertips, it is up to us to help them find ways to feel smart and alert again. We are not saying that we should push people living with dementia or cause them anymore frustration and anxiety than they are already feeling. There is too much fear, frustration, anger and depression in dementia world; we don't need to add to it.

However, we do need to find ways to give people living with dementia a path to being successful again, a way to use their remaining strengths and abilities again. Everyone likes to feel that they are good at something, that they can achieve something, that they can have the right answer, or complete a task. This need to be successful, to feel good about ourselves does not go away because a person has dementia. We have pioneered and created many exercises and games that can help people living with dementia participate in tasks or exercises and be successful. We will share the exercises that we have created and field tested. You know the person you love better than anyone, and you know what will grab their attention and interest and what won't work at all. Once you see how the tools that we use can work with the person you love, then we encourage you to create your own games, tools, exercises to keep the person you care for engaged, active, successful for as long as you can. This is a gift for the person you love and a gift for you, too.

GUIDEPOST:

We all like to be successful, to feel that we can accomplish a task or know the right answer.

The last part of the declarative memory system that is affected by dementia is executive function. Executive function is the ability to plan, the ability to begin an activity, or stop an activity. At its highest level, executive function is what we use when we set goals for ourselves, begin long term projects, and decide on life courses. Executive function helps us understand that our actions have consequences. At its more basic and simple level, executive function helps us understand the order of steps needed to perform simple tasks, such as making coffee, making a peanut butter and jelly sandwich, or getting dressed in the morning. You can see from this list that the role of executive function is huge in our lives. When this part of the memory system is affected, people find it very difficult to carry out the simple, basic tasks of everyday living. This is when we often see people leaving little notes for themselves, reminders of how to perform simple tasks, or reminders of where they parked the car, how to use the telephone, etc. These are often the first clues to family members that the person they love is struggling with memory function.

Think about how difficult life becomes when you can't remember how to begin the first step of so many activities. What if you couldn't remember how to button your shirt? When you stop and analyze this activity, it can become quite involved. There are many steps to buttoning a shirt. What would the first one be? Interestingly, when we ask people who don't have dementia to begin a simple task, such as buttoning a shirt, making a peanut butter and jelly sandwich, loading a washing machine with dirty clothes, we always, always, get different answers from different people. Everyone has their own way of buttoning a shirt, making a sandwich and loading a washer.

For instance, what do you pick up first when you start to make a sandwich? Visualize this in your mind: is it the bread, the knife, the jar of peanut butter? Our point is that even the most simple, mundane, daily task can seem difficult and overwhelming if you can't remember how to start, if you no longer know where to begin. This failure to initiate, this inability to begin a task is the point where many people with dementia begin to give up. They don't know where to start, so they don't start. It is our job as caregivers to help them find a way to begin again.

Betty's Story:

Betty was a person who found that she could no longer remember how to begin the simple tasks of daily living. Because of this failure of executive function, she began to scale back her life and her activities. Betty still lived in the home where she had raised her five children. She had loved to cook and have the family over for big Sunday dinners. Her daughters were shocked when their mother called them up and told them that she didn't want them coming over on Sundays anymore, it was all too much for her. They could hear the emotion, the near panic in their mother's voice. As time went on, their mother became more withdrawn, less active, and began to sleep through much of the day, staying awake most of the night.

The family was finally able to get Betty to the doctor, where they were not surprised to hear that their mother was dealing with dementia, probably Alzheimer's. She was still able to live in her own home, but she just wasn't 'mom' anymore. As time went on, the family noticed that Betty was losing weight and seemed tired all of the time. She was becoming argumentative, refused company and would often not answer her phone. At this time, Betty's daughters were becoming very worried about their mother and her health in general. One of the daughters finally decided to have an honest talk with her mother and discuss future plans.

As they sat across the kitchen table from each other, Betty's daughter realized how cold and sterile the kitchen seemed. This room had been the heart of the house, with something always bubbling on the stove or baking in the oven. Betty's daughter began by asking her mother the big question,

"Mom, what do you want us to do? You can't live here anymore. You know that you aren't doing well. Do you want to live with one of us, or take turns living with some of us, or do you want to go into an assisted living apartment? We want you to help us make this decision. We want you to tell us what you want."

Betty seemed to understand what her daughter was saying to her, but instead of answering any of the life changing questions put before her, Betty simply said,

"I want to know where my things are."

Betty's daughter was dumbfounded. She had no idea what her mother was talking about.

Betty began to cry,

"I don't know where any of my things are. Where are my pots and pans? Where are my spoons?"

Betty's daughter looked around the kitchen, at the gleaming, empty counter tops, the closed cabinets, the shut drawers. Suddenly, she realized that Betty didn't know where her cooking things were because she couldn't see them. Betty didn't remember where anything was and she didn't remember how to open the cabinets and the drawers to find the things she needed.

With her daughter by her side, they began to open drawers, fling open cabinets. Betty looked lovingly at her newly found things, but her daughter knew that she would soon forget where everything was. To help give her mother some immediate relief, Betty's daughter made signs for all of the cabinets and drawers, listing the tools, dishes, cups, pots and pans found behind each closed cabinet, each shut drawer. Everyone knew that this was just a short term aid for their mother while they researched a more lasting solution to their mother's needs.

While they took their mother to visit assisted living places, they also wrote out recipe cards for her to follow so that she could once again make some of her favorite meals. All of the daughters pitched in, making cards with the steps for washing clothes, making coffee, getting dressed. They wrote out directions step by step and taped the cards in the appropriate places. Their mother began to gain weight, to become more social, to seem more like her old self.

The family knew that taping up cards with the steps to simple tasks was not the long term answer their mother needed, but they saw that their mother was regaining some of her independence and some of the joy in her life. She could once again make a visitor a cup of coffee or bake cookies for her grandchildren. These everyday tasks gave Betty great happiness and gave her family real joy. They still had the large decisions to make as a family, but in the meantime, the family had helped Betty find a way to continue to do those things that made her such a special person.

GUIDEPOST:

Failure to initiate is not failure.

The declarative memory system can be greatly affected by dementia but it does not mean that the person we love is no longer the person we love. We have to find new paths to reach them, new ways to engage them, new techniques to help them maintain their strengths and abilities for as long as possible. We all like to feel that we can be successful, that we have something positive to contribute, even when we are living with dementia.

CHAPTER THREE:
I Want to Hold Your Hand

WHILE THE DECLARATIVE memory system controls language, recent events, facts and executive function, there is another memory system that also plays a large role in the life of a person living with Alzheimer's: the procedural memory system. This is the system that controls repetitive muscle memory. Think of riding a bike, swimming, reading, playing a musical instrument, any activity that you learned to do through repetitive movement. The procedural memory system tends to be less affected by dementia. This is why a person with dementia might still be able to play the piano, remember the lyrics to songs, recite memorized poetry or prayers, play cards, or remember how to play baseball. All of these activities call on muscle movement.

We may not have gone swimming for thirty years, but once we hit the water, our bodies remember how to swim. We may not have played the violin for years, but we still know how to play,

GUIDEPOST:

The procedural memory system (muscle memory) tends to be less affected by dementia.

perhaps even remembering a song memorized for a recital when we were twelve years old. We might be rusty, but we still remember how to play. And of course, we've all heard the old adage that you never forget how to ride a bike. Well, it's true, once you learn how to ride a bike, you never forget, even if you are in your eighties and haven't been on a bike since you were ten years old. Your body remembers. This ability to remember through our bodies (muscle memory) is astonishing! Understanding the power of procedural or muscle memory is very helpful in planning a care program for people living with dementia.

There are ways to help prime the pump of memory using techniques that we have pioneered to help people find new ways to be successful. One of the most effective techniques we use to prime the pump of memory is also one of the most simple: put something meaningful in a person's hands.

Debbie's Story:

Debbie was a small, wiry woman we met while we were working in a locked dementia unit. Debbie was the community scourge; she was constantly going into other people's rooms and taking things that did not belong to her. She was very bossy and argumentative. She would say hurtful things to people, both residents and staff. Her family was embarrassed by her behavior, often apologizing and telling us that this behavior was not at all like their mother; their mother had been the soul of politeness and was well liked in her neighborhood and church. They could not understand Debbie's aggressive attitude and her constant pilfering.

Debbie's family told us that she had loved flowers and was known as the "flower lady" of their small town. Based on this knowledge of her personal interests, we decided to bring in real flowers and some vases for Debbie to do flower arranging. We also brought a pitcher with water so that she could fill the vases with water for the flowers. When Debbie saw the flowers, she rushed up to them and snatched them up in her arms, holding them against her chest with a look of challenge in her eyes. We told Debbie that we brought the flowers for her to arrange for the dining room tables.

Instead of using the safety scissors that we brought for Debbie, she began to break the stems in her hands. Crack, crack, crack, the ends of the flower stems flew all over the dining room as Debbie worked feverishly, arranging the roses, lilies and daisies in various vases. As time went on, Debbie began to work more slowly, with more care. She would turn the vases to see if the flower arrangements were balanced. She carefully poured the water into the vases; if some spilled, she wiped up the spilled water. A sense of calm and purpose came over Debbie as she worked with the flowers. When she finished the task, Debbie had a table filled with beautifully arranged flowers, each arrangement different, and each lovely. We asked Debbie if she would like to put the flowers on the dining room tables. At first, she hesitated, but then she told us,

"That lady who sits there (pointing at a table) likes roses. I will give her this one with all of the roses."

Debbie became the flower lady again, this time the flower lady of the dementia unit. She still had problems with pilfering pretty things from other people's rooms, but her attitude began to change. She may not have remembered that she was the person responsible for the beautiful flower arrangements in the dining room, but she loved looking at the flowers every day. We think that somewhere, deep inside, Debbie did know that she was once again making a meaningful contribution to her community by providing their dining room with her special flower arrangements.

Through the years, as we have worked in retirement communities, adult day centers and memory clinics, we have discovered some simple but powerful tools for engaging people who are living with dementia. One of the first ideas that we broach when we are consulting with families or training staff is this one very simple thing: put something meaningful in a person's hands.

This meaningful object can be something that the person loved, or it could be something from nature, or it could be a small sculpture or a beautiful photograph.

We all have a bond with nature, even those of us who live in cities. There is a resonance when we hold something made of wood; the wood takes on the warmth of our hands. Even something as common as a smooth stone can take on special meaning when placed in the hands of a person living with Alzheimer's. Leaves, flowers, a cup of snow can bring forth a torrent of memories for elders who are now living in locked dementia units, or who rarely venture outside.

GAME:
PENNANT SORT

Once we understand the importance of giving people something to hold, the exercises and activities we can create are limited only by our own imagination. Perhaps the person you care for loved baseball. Obviously, a baseball or baseball mitt, a baseball pennant or cap of their favorite team can be an excellent way to bring back baseball memories and spark conversation. We created a very interesting game by dividing miniature baseball pennants into the teams that belonged to the National League and those teams belonging to the American League. For a baseball fan, this game provides lots of memories and lots of fun. These small pennants can be found and purchased on the Internet. (*see figure 1*)

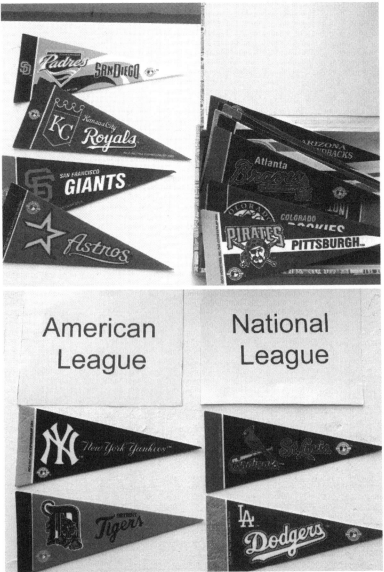

figure 1 - Pennant matching exercise. Using pennants, organize by league to stimulate conversation and memory.

GAME:
TACKLE BOX

Another exercise we created was to fill a tackle box full of matching fishing lures (hooks removed). We also placed matching photographs of fish and pictures of people fishing in the tackle box. We have spent many hours with this tackle box, talking to both men and women about their memories of fishing and the big ones who got away.

GAME:
FABRIC MATCH

Another simple but meaningful exercise is to give people swatches of material to hold in each hand. (*see* **figure 2**) One swatch might be corduroy, another could be satin. These materials feel very different from each other and may bring up memories of wearing certain clothes or even making clothes. We have created lively discussions by bringing in works of art, both paintings and small sculptures. For those people who have trouble with their vision, small sculptures or textured material, real fruits

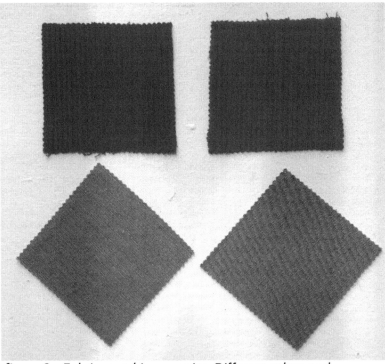

figure 2 - *Fabric matching exercise. Different colors and textures.*

and vegetables are all objects that people can identify from touch or smell.

We build a bridge to the person living with dementia by the simple act of placing a meaningful object in their hands. For people living with dementia, it can be very difficult to begin a conversation or spark memories from thin air. Giving people things to hold that are from nature, or from their own life experience, is a powerful way to help connect elders to the larger world again.

Sam's Story:

Sam's mother had been a talented violinist. As she passed through the final stage of Alzheimer's, her family could not find any way to connect with her. She rarely opened her eyes to look at them, and never had any reaction to seeing them. She offered no smiles and no look of recognition. Sam was near tears when he contacted us and asked for our help. The family knew, of course, that their mother was near death, but they wanted to be able to feel that they were with her in these last days.

GUIDEPOST:

Put something meaningful in their hands.

Knowing his mother's history, we encouraged Sam to place his mother's violin in her hands[3], even as she lay with her eyes closed. We also asked him to play some CD's of his mother's favorite music. Sam told us that when he placed his mother's violin in her hands, her eyes flew open and she began to stroke the beloved instrument. For the first time in months, Sam's mother looked at him and smiled. The last few days of Sam's mother's life were spent listening to her favorite music, her violin in her arms, and her family with her to the end.

---

[3] Author's Note: Please make sure that the objects you use are safe: too large to be swallowed, nothing sharp or pointed, and nothing toxic.

Henry's Story:

Henry had been diagnosed with early onset Alzheimer's (when symptoms of Alzheimer's begin before the age of 65) and was living in a memory enhancement center. He was a very quiet, withdrawn man, not easy to draw into conversation. The staff told us that Henry had been a serious collector of vintage cars. With this information in mind, we went to an automobile junk yard and searched for hub caps from vintage cars. We took the hub caps with some non-toxic metal polish and cloths to the center where Henry was living. We invited Henry to help us polish the hub caps. (figure 3) He agreed to work with us. We started talking about the Studebaker hub caps and their unique design. Henry didn't reply, he just kept diligently polishing the hub caps. We sat in silence, working on the hub caps together.

After some time, Henry started talking quietly about his time as a soldier in Viet Nam. He spoke from the heart, with a lot of emotion about his time in the war. We were stunned; we never expected this sort of reminiscence from Henry, who seemed so remote and withdrawn. On reflection, we thought that perhaps the motion of polishing brought up memories for Henry of polishing his boots or his brass before an inspection in the army. This simple exercise helped Henry release some powerful emotions and memories. He would have never opened up this way if we had sat down and said to him, "Okay, Henry. Tell us about some of your experiences in Viet Nam."

Henry would have probably looked at us blankly and walked away from us, feeling angry or depressed that we had demanded information from him that he could not access, or did not want to access. In order to have a relationship with people living with dementia, we need some way to bridge the gap, some way to prime the pump of conversation and of memory. Engaging the procedural memory system is one way we have found that is very successful in helping us reach people with dementia and engage them in meaningful work, and meaningful conversation.

Our experience with Henry reminded us how important it is to follow the lead of the person we are working with.

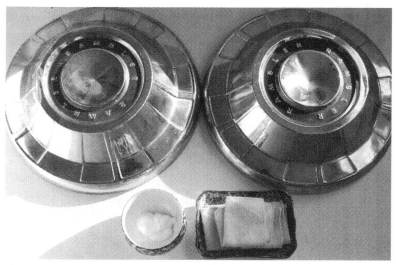

figure 3 - *Hubcap polishing exercise.*

We thought Henry might want to talk about his

collection of vintage cars, but he wanted to share his memories of Viet Nam. The lesson we learned from Henry is that once we make a connection, we never know where it will lead. Staying connected to a person with dementia means that we need to be prepared to go with the flow. We may have had certain plans for Henry, but in that moment it was important to put our ideas and plans aside and listen to the memories he was able to share; to appreciate this experience of connecting with him. We have learned so much and had so many profound experiences in this memory support work when we were able to let go and simply follow.

Once we understand how important it is to engage people through their hands, we are only limited by our own imagination. We should not only think about what a person did for a living when we are developing meaningful experiences for them, we should think about what their interests and passions were. A man may have been a plumber all of his life, but that does not necessarily mean that we should give him pipes and wrenches. Maybe he didn't like being a plumber, or maybe he grew tired of working with wrenches and pipes. Perhaps model trains or college football were his real interests. That is why we have to find out what people really liked to do, what their passions are, and their true interests. Sometimes, the answers are really surprising!

Glen's Story:

We experienced one of these surprises one day when we met with Glen, a PhD from a prestigious university. He had spent his life learning and teaching philosophy and theology. Glen was furious that his family had placed him in a locked care center. His family reported that he had grown more and more difficult to care for at home as his dementia grew worse. Glen began to sleep all day and stay awake at night, sometimes trying to drive off in the car. His wife was exhausted and at her wits' end when the family decided that Glen needed more professional help than they could provide for him at home. Glen was very loud in his complaints about his living conditions in the care center, and was often abusive to his family when they came to visit. Most of the staff gave Glen a wide berth because they found his constant criticisms hard to take day after day.

We were familiar with the university where Glen received his PhD and so he would often talk to us about the campus and the neighborhood around the university. Even though Glen was willing to talk with us, he always refused to participate in any of the work that we brought to the care facility where he was living. He would tell us,

"I know what you are up to, and it is no good. There is nothing you can do to help me, there is nothing anyone can do to help." We never argued with Glen. We acknowledged his feelings and honored his wishes.

One day, in the middle of summer, we brought in bunches of fresh herbs from our garden to the care center where Glen was living. We brought the herbs for a gardening group that we had started at the center. We tied up pairs of herbs with green ribbon so that the people in the group could match the herbs, either by sight, scent, or touch. We had bundles of sage, thyme, rosemary, lavender, and mint. We also brought card stock and markers, so that people could make labels for the herbs as they matched pairs of them.

A small group gathered around the table, picking up the herbs, smelling them, rubbing the soft, green leaves between their fingers. Suddenly, we noticed that Glen had joined the group of people at the table. He picked up a bunch of sage and rubbed the green, velvety leaves against his cheek and sniffed deeply. Glen began to softly sing,

"Are you going to Scarborough Fair? Parsley, sage, rosemary and thyme."

We were astonished that Glen was so taken with the herbs and that he would burst into song. He had always seemed such a hard boiled, coldly intellectual person. Glen then went on to tell us about his mother, who had a large herb garden and collected heirloom seeds for her garden. Glen told us the story of how he, as a little boy, had found his mother's precious stash of heirloom seeds and proceeded to scatter the seeds all over the farm. He laughed as he remembered the plants growing in the oddest places that spring and summer.

"We had peas and rhubarb growing in the outhouse!"

Even though we had spent many hours talking with Glen, we would have never guessed that herbs would have unlocked so many wonderful memories for him.

For the time, Glen seemed genuinely happy that summer day as he rubbed the herbs between his fingers and remembered his mother's garden.

When we hold one of our training seminars, people are often surprised to learn how powerful it can be when we do this one simple thing, when we put something meaningful in a person's hand. Ryan, an administrator of a long term care center, attended one of our trainings and raised an objection as we were explaining this simple but powerful tool. He was a highly educated person, well versed on the latest research in dementia and very interested in our work. He was also quite young, in his twenties. It is unusual to find someone this young working as an administrator of a large nursing home. We were demonstrating the use of objects from nature and had brought in matching stones to show the class. These were smooth river stones (too large for people with dementia to try and swallow but not too heavy for them to comfortably hold). We pointed out the satisfaction that comes from the simple act of holding these types of stones in the hand; the stones are smooth to the touch, they take on the warmth of the human hand when held for a while and they were different shapes and colors. Ryan's objection to this exercise was that he could not see himself, when he was an old man, sitting around holding different types of rocks in his hands.

One of the other attendees of our training class was the polar opposite of Ryan. He was an older man who had spent years in the aging field. He smiled warmly at Ryan and told him,

"Son, these stones have had all of their rough edges worn off by the flow of water over them for years and years. People my age and older know what it feels like to have life knock off some of our rough edges. Believe me, when you are an old guy like me, you will understand the lessons that these stones teach us."

We were the trainers, the teachers of this class, but that day we learned a very valuable lesson from one of our students. We have learned so much (and continue to learn every day) in this dementia work. From Debbie (the flower lady) we learned the importance of remaining a contributing member of one's community, from Glen (the professor) we learned that nature can touch even the most intellectual person, and from Henry (the vintage car collector) we learned that sometimes polishing hubcaps is much more than polishing hubcaps!

CHAPTER FOUR:

Come Together

IN OUR WORK, we try and create meaningful moments, fleeting times of connection in order to stay in relationship with the person who is living with dementia. We know that our work cannot bring the person back to the way they were before they had dementia, we know that these connections may come and go in a flash, we know that these moments of connection cannot change the condition of the person living with dementia, nor can these fleeting moments change the pain and loneliness of the people who love them. So, why even bother? Why rack our brains for ideas, why create special things for people to hold or taste or look at? If it all comes down to just a couple of minutes of recognition or a moment of connection, is it worth the work, the effort?

To answer that question, we have to take a look at our own lives. When you think about it, all of us live our lives in fleeting moments; we nod and smile at someone at work, we give a quick kiss to the people we love, we catch a glimpse of a beautiful sunset, we hear a much loved song on the radio. Our own lives are lived moment by moment. Our own memories are fleeting as well. We remember snatches of a conversation, a scene from the past, a familiar gesture, the taste of a favorite food. We, whose memory and mind may still be strong, are able to hold long conversations, sit through a two-hour movie, or read an entire book. But what do we, with our intact memory systems, remember from these events? If we are lucky, we remember the general topic of a conversation, a few scenes from the movie, and the theme of the book. All of us, those who live with dementia and those of us who do not live with dementia, all of us live our lives moment by moment. When we try to connect to those of us who have dementia, we are doing something that is not so very different from the way we live our own lives.

We just need to be more conscious of the immediacy and the momentary nature of life when we reach out to people living with dementia. Living in the moment is not a bad way to approach life. This moment is, after all, the only time we have. With our intact memory systems and our highly functioning cognitive abilities, we tend to race from one event to the next. People living with dementia teach us the importance of slowing down. They teach us an essential lesson: there is only *this* moment in time.

We had this lesson brought home to us on a warm summer afternoon as we sat under the umbrellas of a sidewalk restaurant watching the world stroll by. Next to our table was a young family, mom and dad and two little boys. While the boys savored their handmade ice cream cones, we couldn't help but notice that both of their parents were completely immersed in their hand held devices. Both parents had their eyes cast downwards, not looking at their children or each other, staring fixedly at the small screens in their hands. This moment: the lovely summer sky, the colorful people walking by, the yellow and green umbrellas of the restaurant, the flower boxes in full bloom on the sidewalk railings, the ice cream, and the little boys' enraptured faces, were all lost on the two people staring into their handheld devices.

We live in a marvelous age of great leaps in technology, almost a renaissance period of change and growth. But if we surrender moments of engagement, moments of relationships to this technology, we will begin to lose pieces of our lives. These moments are usually just ordinary things, a family dinner, a run by the lake, a child in our arms, but these are the moments that matter; these are the moments that make up our lives.

When we were parents of young children, it was hard to make the time (even five minutes) to just talk to our children one on one and to really, really listen. Yet those five minutes, those quiet talks, those little moments are how we build and grow relationships, memories, our lives. People living with dementia teach us to pay attention. They remind us to look at the faces of the people we love, to really listen to the music in our life, feel the wind on our face, taste the ice cream. These moments are the jewels of our lives strung on the necklace of time.

GUIDEPOST:

The eternal NOW.

We are not saying that dementia is a good thing. We fully realize the pain and suffering that this condition causes. We are saying that the people who live with dementia can still be teachers, can still share wisdom, humor, stories, and compassion, if we are willing to make the effort it takes to reach them. It is not easy to make the connection with someone who stares right through you, who doesn't remember who you are, or perhaps, doesn't even acknowledge your presence. We understand how difficult this is. We can only imagine the pain of sitting by someone you have loved for years (perhaps your entire life) and they don't have a clue who you are. We know that dementia is hard, dementia is painful, and dementia is lonely. We also know that as long as the person you love is alive, you do a great service to them and to yourself when you try and connect to them, however you can. We know, too, that these moments of engagement are fleeting, just as all of the moments of our lives are fleeting.

Philosophers and theologians of all persuasions and belief systems have discussed at length this concept of living life in the moment. Paul Tillich, a German theologian and philosopher, called this approach to life, "the eternal now." He writes this of the eternal now,

"In the present, our future and our past are *ours*."

GUIDEPOST:

These feelings of warmth are like anchors in our lives.

How do we keep the future and the past *ours* with someone who has dementia? We want so much for our loved ones to remember everything we remember. We feel like our memories are the ties that bind us together. It is lonely and sad when the person you love can no longer share specific events or important occasions with you.

These feelings of warmth are like an anchor in our lives; we cannot always delineate these memories point by point, day by day, but nevertheless, we have this anchor, this center that runs deeply through our lives. People who live with memory loss experience the breaking of some of the links to this anchor, but the center still holds. We are trying to find the links to help people with memory loss reconnect this chain, link by link, moment by moment.

We want to shout at them that they must remember! How could they forget? When someone you love no longer remembers a shared event, it is as though they are rejecting us, as though our shared life no longer matters to them. When we're feeling this way, it is important to consider the nature of the dementia condition and how it affects the memory and cognitive ability. Even though it is very difficult, we have to push through the sadness and loneliness we feel and make a grand effort to reach the person we love. Our goal must be to come together, even for a moment, even if it is just holding hands, or sharing a smile, or crying together.

Over the years of working with people who live with dementia, we have learned how to celebrate the smallest of victories, the tiniest step, and the fleeting breakthroughs. When someone with dementia recognizes our face (even though they don't remember our name) it is time to break out the champagne, blow up balloons and have a party! We have learned how to appreciate so many small moments in this work. This celebratory attitude has spilled over into our own lives; we have learned to appreciate so many small moments in our own lives at home with our family.

We need to learn how to walk through this dementia life. Have you ever been on a walk with a toddler? A walk that would take an adult twenty minutes to complete can take a toddler two hours! It is not just that they have much shorter legs, and are much more unsteady on their feet, the reality is that toddlers don't walk to get to a destination. Toddlers walk for the sheer joy of movement and the sheer joy of seeing the world around them. Have you noticed how they stop and study the smallest things? Even an ant on the sidewalk deserves the full attention of a two year old. We can find many more moments of joy traveling through the dementia experience if we take our time, just as a toddler moves down the sidewalk, noticing everything, taking joy in the smallest thing, being fascinated by the ordinary, celebrating it all!

We were once in a waiting room and watched the interaction of a mother with her little girl. The little girl was about five years old and absolutely enthralled with the pigeons pecking away just outside the window of the waiting room. She was telling her mother how beautiful she thought the white pigeon was when her mother replied,

"Oh, those old pigeons are like flying rats. They are so dirty and full of germs!"

We saw the little girl's face fall and she moved away from the window, turning her back on the pigeons.

Well, of course, her mother was right, pigeons aren't the cleanest of birds, but her little girl was right, too. That white pigeon was very beautiful. We have to check ourselves when we interact with young children and with elders. Are we trying to see the world through their eyes? Or are we ignoring them? Very young children and people living with dementia have a lot in common. It is not that people with dementia are child- like or infantile. Older people deserve to be treated with the full measure of respect and dignity that they have earned. The point where children and people with dementia intersect is at the crossroads of wonder. People with dementia have lost a lot, but they still have their curiosity, their ability to feel wonder.

Again, if we willing to learn this lesson, people living

with dementia can teach us how to feel wonder again at very small moments, seemingly insignificant events. We have to be willing to slow down, to breathe deeply, and to pay attention to this moment. We were working in a memory enhancement center, helping the staff deal with sundowning (the wandering behavior in the evening or night time hours that often occurs with people who have dementia). The administrator of this center invited us to spend some evenings in their dementia unit to work with the staff on developing end of day activities for the people living there. We developed some poetry reading circles, and some singing circles, and found that these groups helped the older people to find some sense of calm and some sense of community as their day came to an end.

Dale's Story:

We were leaving this memory enhancement center one night when one of the residents stopped us. Dale had been a farmer before he came to live in the dementia unit. He wanted to talk to us about his life on the farm. He was very proud of his 4020 John Deere tractor that had thousands of hours logged on it. Dale spoke of this tractor as though it were a living creature. One of the exercises that we developed for this rural facility was matching pairs of photos of tractors. As Dale talked to us about his beloved tractor, we took out some photos of tractors that we had brought with us that day. One of the photos was of a tractor parked in high grass. We mentioned to Dale that this tractor looked like it had seen better days and was probably no longer working. Dale shook his head at us and said,

"No, the tractor probably isn't broken; it's just parked in high grass. It's an old machine, alright, but she's probably got some good days in her yet. Sometimes, you have to look deeper to see what is really going on."

That night, Dale died in his sleep. We may have been the last people to whom he ever spoke. Even then, at the very end of his life, Dale taught us a life lesson that we have never forgotten.

We learned to take the time to really look, to try and really see, to truly understand the picture before we judge what is going on.

We know that this approach to dementia is not part of the common discussion around this condition. We realize that some people may be angered by our belief that people living with dementia have important life lessons to teach us. We understand that some people are so angry, or so despondent about dementia that they cannot believe us when we say that there can be beautiful and touching moments in this experience. We do appreciate these emotions, but we also know what we ourselves have experienced over and over again in this work.

GUIDEPOST:

We have met many different kinds of people living with dementia and all of them have this one thing in common: There is not a phony in the bunch!

We meet people who don't know what year it is, who are not sure where they are, or what they are doing now. They also don't seem to care much about the kind of car we drive, or our politics, or our religious beliefs. They don't care how much money we have, how big our house is, how expensive our clothes are, or what college we attended. When these people living with dementia connect with us, they connect with us soul to soul. Everything superficial falls away, and we see the essence of the person. They are not angelic people, many have mean streaks, or a wicked sense of humor or they may be depressed or touchy, bad tempered and difficult. They may also be extraordinarily kind, or curious, or joyful or very, very funny. We have met many different kinds of people living with dementia, and all of them have this one thing in common: there is not a phony in the bunch! They are truly, completely themselves without pretense, without apology.

It is a wonderful gift to be in the presence of people who

no longer feel the need to pretend or be hypocritical. It is refreshing to have a connection with people who are completely honest and completely their essential selves. They have no agenda, they don't play games, they speak their truth and share their true feelings. It is an honor to be in the presence of those for whom all has fallen away, for whom this moment is the only moment, for whom the wonder of small things is very real.

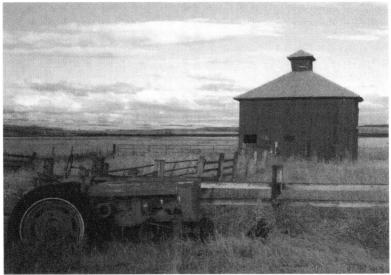

Photo by Jay W. Krajic.

CHAPTER FIVE:
The Word

WE HAVE LEARNED over the years to look for the strengths and spared abilities in people living with dementia. One of the abilities that we count as strength is the ability to read. Many people living with dementia (even those in the last stages of this condition) are still able to read. Sometimes, elders say that they can no longer read when what they really mean is that they cannot see smaller print. If we produce reading material in large enough print then many people can still read. There are, of course, some people who lose the ability to read. For those people, we recommend that the reading materials we have created be read aloud to them. We often suggest that people with dementia read aloud to their fellow residents who can no longer read. Or, we may encourage reading aloud to a young child. These spared abilities and strengths can be used as a means to give back to the community where the person with dementia is living, whether that community is an intentional one, as in a long term care center, or a family home.

Even though we count reading as a great strength, if a person can't remember what he read five minutes ago, does reading still hold value for that person? Would this experience be frustrating to a person with dementia? We don't recommend that people be given entire books to read, or even an entire magazine or newspaper. Instead, we have developed materials for reading that are a better fit for people living with dementia. These materials address the memory deficits as well as the interests and abilities of older people.

Understanding that people with dementia are dealing with memory loss and cognitive difficulties, we have created materials that are short, to the point and written in large enough print for the individual reader. We incorporate simple poems, very short stories, songs, hymns, prayers and jokes in our reading program. Our reading program is based on the interests of the people with whom we are working. We discovered that heartfelt emotion, humor and word games are important tools to engage people.

We will begin by describing how we use poetry to reach people living with dementia. We have used the poetry of all sorts of poets, from Wordsworth to Ciardi to amateur poets who very kindly shared their work with us. We spent several years working at a home for elderly Scandinavian Americans. One bitterly cold winter afternoon, we brought in a stanza from Wordsworth's *Prelude:*

And in the frosty season, when the sun
Was set, and visible for many a mile
The cottage windows through the twilight blazed,
I heeded not their summons. Clear and loud
The village clock tolled six; I wheeled about
Proud and exulting, like an untired horse
That cares not for his home. All shod with steel
We hissed along the polished ice in games...

Not seldom from the uproar I retired
Into a silent bay, or sportively
Glanced sideway, leaving the tumultuous throng,
To cut across the shadow of a star
That gleamed upon the ice. And oftentimes
When we had given our bodies to the wind,
And all the shadowy banks on either side
Came sweeping through the darkness, spinning still
The rapid line of motion, then at once
Have I, reclining back upon my heels,
Stopped short --- yet still the solitary cliffs
Wheeled by me...

The language in this poem is not easy, but the people we asked to read that day seemed to really enjoy the poem We were wondering if they truly understood the poem, when one of the residents rose slowly from her chair, leaned forward and put her arms straight back behind her.

"That's how you catch the wind when you're skating. That way you can go really, really fast!" This group obviously understood the poem and it sparked wonderful memories of skating when they were children. Sometimes, if the interest is great, people will rise to the challenge of a more difficult poem. While it is important to try very hard not to frustrate people who are already dealing with so many difficulties, it is equally important to give people the chance to stretch a little, to reach a little.

> # GUIDEPOST:
>
> While it is important to try very hard not to frustrate people who are already dealing with so many difficulties, it is equally important to give the chance to stretch a little, to reach a little.

We print the poems in large font and put them in notebooks with the name of the poet on the front. Older people who studied poetry when they were young respond very deeply to the rhythm and meter of poetry. We have often been surprised by the emotion and drama that some people will bring to reading poetry aloud. Reading poetry was part of almost everyone's education in earlier generations and the people we work with often become very animated and engaged when reading poetry aloud together.

When we began creating poetry reading circles for people with dementia, some surprising things began to happen: people began to give us poetry written by their aunts, or husbands, or their own personal poetry. We have been given poetry by people living on farms and in cities, written by older people, younger people, and people of all descriptions. Some of these poems are more polished than others, but all of them strike a chord with the people who read them aloud. These homespun poems often bring up some vivid memories and lively conversations. Here is one example of the poetry that has been shared with us:

The Girl in the Picture
-Evelyn Grisso Pittenger

Today, high on a closet shelf
I found an old picture of myself

When I was young, pretty and slim,
And filled with energy, vigor and vim.

I looked at the picture in my hand
And tried my best to understand
How could this pretty lissome lass
Be the woman I see in my looking glass?

She had her dreams, this girl that was me.
But the woman I am has my memories.
The girl in the picture has youth on her side,
While I have a waistline I try to hide.

The girl in the picture is happy, no doubt.
But she doesn't know what life's all about.
While I've gathered memories along life's way,
To make me the woman I am today.

This poem evokes a lot of talk about many different topics; from the aging process to teen age memories, dances, boyfriends, schools. There is something so simple, heartfelt and genuine in this poem.

Many of this older generation had to memorize poetry as part of their education. Some people still remember entire poems or a few lines of poetry from their school days. Almost all of the people of this generation have a deep love for poetry and an understanding of this art form that younger generations don't share. Still, we were sometimes surprised by some of the people we met who loved poetry.

Gerry's Story:

Gerry was a tough customer, a woman who had been a professional truck driver at a time when women were not often found in this profession. Gerry terrorized the dementia unit where she was living. She would hit people, throw things across the room and curse out the staff when they annoyed her. One day we were working on a puzzle with Gerry when she spontaneously began to read the words on the puzzle box. When we told the staff that we heard Gerry reading, they were as shocked as we were. She had never joined our reading groups, never picked up a newspaper or magazine, so it was assumed that she could no longer read.

The next shock came when Gerry decided to join one of our poetry reading groups. We would have never guessed that she would be drawn to poetry. Once we realized that Gerry could read and that she enjoyed reading aloud to others, we had the staff ask her to read aloud on a regular basis. We would often walk in and see Gerry surrounded by a group of residents and staff all listening intently while Gerry read poetry to them. The staff told us that once Gerry became the designated reader of the dementia unit, her outbursts of violence and cursing were greatly decreased. She would still roll by in her wheelchair and give us the occasional sharp pinch on our bottoms, but everyone could see the change in Gerry. She loved the poems and she loved reading aloud to others.

Ava's Story:

As we learned with Gerry, there were many people who surprised us with their ability to read. From Ava, we learned to always give people a chance, no matter how difficult the circumstances. We met Ava when she was living in the infirmary of a long term care center. Ava had come to the facility when she was diagnosed with Alzheimer's; while there, she had a stroke that left her paralyzed on one side, with the use of only one eye. We were surprised when the staff member wheeled Ava up to the table for our reading circle. She was slumped over with a patch on one eye, barely able to lift her head.

*We passed out the notebooks with the short, funny stories and jokes that we had printed in large font. (see **figure 4**) We looked at each other briefly, wondering if we should hand the book to Ava, but before we could decide, Ava put out her hand and took the book from us. Everyone took a turn reading the stories and jokes out loud. There were soft chuckles and some guffaws as the humorous stories and corny jokes were read by each of the elders. We heard a dry sort of cackle and realized that Ava was laughing, too. Finally, it was Ava's turn to read and we held our breath, wondering what would happen.*

She held the book with her one good hand and turned her head to see the print with her one good eye. Ava started out hesitatingly, in a small, cracked little voice; but as she began to get into the jokes she was reading, her voice picked up strength and expression. The more she read, the better she became at reading. Everything in the infirmary just stopped; the nurses and aides all stood very still, even the aide mopping the floor stopped and leaned on her mop to listen to Ava read. Sitting up straighter in her wheelchair, and with a strong voice, Ava read the last joke:

"What did the bra say to the top hat?"

She waited just a tick (as would any good comedienne) and fixed her audience with her one good eye. Then came the punch line,
"You go on a head. I'll give these two a lift!"

As the crowd around the table chuckled, Ava handed us the book of jokes and said,

"Now that was funny!"

Ava taught us to never give up on anyone, to always try, to always give everyone a chance.

GUIDEPOST:

We learned to always give people a chance, no matter how difficult the circumstances.

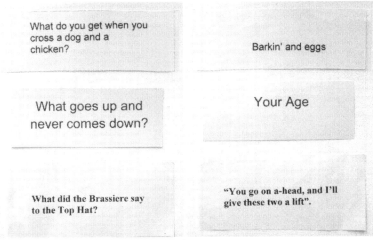

What do you get when you cross a dog and a chicken?

Barkin' and eggs

What goes up and never comes down?

Your Age

What did the Brassiere say to the Top Hat?

"You go on a-head, and I'll give these two a lift".

figure 4 - Joke Exercise Material

As well as reading poetry and short stories together, we have also created word finding games to play together. As we discussed earlier, having difficulty in finding words is a common occurrence for people living with dementia. Sometimes, people may struggle to find the names of common objects. They may describe the object in detail and yet not be able to come up with the name of the object.

"You know that thing. I need it. You hold it in your hand, and stuff comes out of the end. I use it to write letters."

Obviously, this is a description of a pen or pencil. Sometimes, though, there is a lot of guessing in trying to determine the object that a person with dementia is trying to describe. As frustrating as this process may be for the listener, imagine how frustrating and how frightening this laborious process must be for the person who can't think of the names of the most common of objects. We know the frustration we feel with the tip of the tongue phenomenon. Can you imagine that feeling plaguing you all of the time? It would be exhausting. This inability to name common objects can also extend to the names of people, even people who are very close to the person with dementia.

It is devastating when our mother or husband no longer remembers our name; no longer remembers the life we shared together. From our work in dementia care, we have learned that while people living with dementia may not be able to bring up names or specific memories, they can (and often do) relate to loved ones on a more spiritual level. This is a phenomenon we have noted in people who were deeply religious and those who never practiced any sort of religion. There is a soul to soul connection that we have seen over and over again. Once we get passed the inability to remember names, words, specific memories, we can learn to look for small signs of recognition; the squeezed hand, the fleeting smile, the remembered song.

While it may seem counter intuitive to create word finding games for people who obviously struggle to remember words, we have found that people can get better at these games with time and familiarity.

(Remember the procedural memory system; people can improve when given the opportunity to repeat an activity.) Again, we must strike a balance between frustrating people and giving them a goal to reach for. These games are meant to help improve the ability to find words as well as giving people with dementia the opportunity to be social, have fun and laugh again. The game is a vehicle, a tool for promoting reminiscence, conversation, bonding with others, as well as providing a repetitive exercise for improving word finding skills.

We will give you here two examples of word finding games that have proven to be very successful. These games can be played by large groups, by small groups or with only two people. We have used them in long term care centers, adult day centers, memory enhancement centers and family homes.

GUIDEPOST:

While it may seem counter-intuitive to create word finding games for people who obviously struggle to remember words, we have found that people can get better at these games with time and familiarity.

GAME:
NAME THIS TUNE

For this game, we created cards with 100 size print. We hand out the cards with the last word of a song printed on it. (*see* **figure 5**)The group leader then holds up and reads aloud the first part of a song title. "Let me call you…" The answer, of course, is "sweetheart." This game often leads to spontaneous group sing alongs. This group singing is wonderful for everyone. These songs also often bring up memories and heartfelt conversations. Music is one of the most evocative activities for memory enhancement exercises. They can be songs that were popular when this particular group of people were young, they can be religious hymns, or holiday songs. The group leader should have a cheat sheet with at least the first verse and chorus lyrics written down so that they can help out with the singing. These games also offer opportunities for people in the group to mentor one another, to help each other when one person reads better than another person.

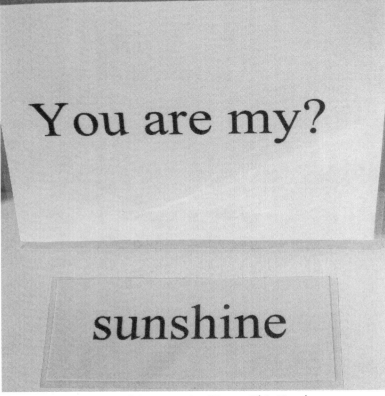

figure 5 - Song-matching exercise 'Name This Tune'.

<u>GAME:</u>
FINISH THE PHRASE

This game is based on the idea of people finishing common sayings or proverbs.

"A stitch in time…"

"Saves nine."

It is astonishing to see people who may say very little, suddenly become very involved in this type of game. These old sayings seem to never leave us. This game is played the same way as the Name that Tune game is played. The group leader holds up the beginning part of the phrase and each participant looks to see if he or she has the final words to the phrase. Again, the purpose is to help people improve their ability to find words, but more importantly, these games promote laughter, engagement and social bonding. It is fun to ask older people what some of these sayings mean, as their original meaning is often lost in the mists of time. What does "the whole nine yards" mean anyway?

GAME:
CATEGORY SORTING
(LIVING/NOT LIVING)

Finally, one other example of word finding games is the game that involves category sorting. We hold different types of objects in different parts of our brain. For example, the word puppy lights up one part of our brain, while the word, screwdriver, lights up another part of our brain. If we can have people think in categories, it is a wonderful way to stimulate the mind.

These categories can be things like "Things we do in winter, things we do in summer." Or, it could be "Things found in a purse, things found in a tool box." We placed a rubber hammer, a screwdriver, pliers, C clamp in a tool box and compact, wallet, comb, tissues in a purse. (*see figure 6*) We made cards with large print stating "Purse" "Tool box." People placed the objects from each under the category they thought best fit the object. If you don't want to use the actual objects, you can just use the printed names that would fit in different categories.

The one category sort exercise that we find to be very successful for people living with dementia is one we call Living/Not Living.

In this exercise we print cards with large font. One card says LIVING on it, one says, NOT LIVING. We place these cards on a table and then bring out cards that describe things that may be living or not living. We try and make these words interesting so that people have to take a moment and think about the exercise. For example, we use words like "rainbow" "wool" "fish."

A fish could be alive or it could be the kind of fish you eat, and therefore, not living. We once had a woman tell us why she put the word "fire truck' in the LIVING column. She said that a fire truck moves fast and it saves lives, so she believed that it belonged in the living category. It's hard to argue with that kind of logic! These sorts of word games are only limited by your imagination. They can be played anywhere by any one.

ACTIVITY:
WORD GAMES/READING

Word games are a wonderful way to reconnect when a family goes to visit a loved one. Or, they are great for bridging the generational divide, having older people play these types of games with younger people or children. The person who is the group leader for these games is also an interesting part of the equation. A group leader could be a nurse, or an aide, or a family member. A group leader could also be someone living with dementia who is able to read and who understands the purpose of the game. We were once beginning a category sort game at a memory enhancement center, when a gentleman asked if he could be the group leader for this game. We were surprised by this request as the man was 102 years old. He did a marvelous job of holding up the signs and reading them aloud and ran the entire game without any help from us, or anyone else!

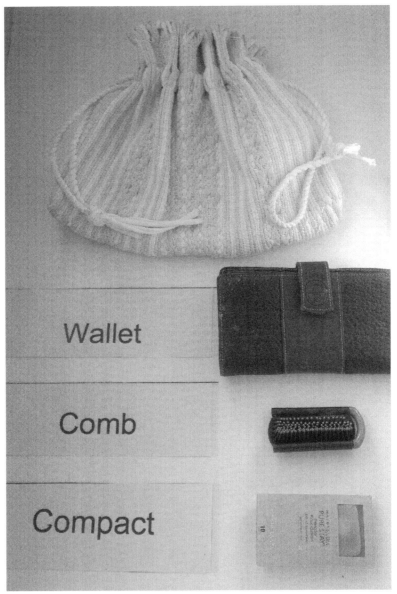

figure 6 - *Category/sorting game.*

One of our most popular reading exercises is our joke reading activity. We use corny jokes with very obvious punch lines. On one side of a card we print in large font the set up for a joke, "What nationality is Santa Claus?"

The punch line is written on the flip side of the card.

The person turns the card over and reads the punch line, "North Polish!" It is so wonderful to see a group of people with dementia laughing together. We were surprised to learn that if we did this joke telling exercise often enough, people would remember to flip the cards over spontaneously without having to be reminded to turn them over for the punch line. We have seen extremely withdrawn people become animated comediennes when we gave them a stack of jokes to read to a group. Everyone gets that warm glow when they are laughing together.

Reading is an activity that uses the procedural memory system (our eyes move back and forth as we read) and is, therefore, often still intact for people living with dementia. For those people who can still read (when the print is large enough) it is vital that we create opportunities for them to practice this spared ability, this remaining skill. Reading can bring great joy to the reader and to the listener. It is a way to help promote better word finding skills as well as creating moments of laughter and moments of engagement. People who struggle with reading can get better, if given the opportunity to read on regular basis. Giving people with dementia the chance to read a poem to others, or to read a funny joke and hear laughter is an experience not to be squandered.

CHAPTER SIX:
In my Life

WHEN WE BEGAN creating short stories for people living with dementia to read aloud, we were surprised by the journey that this simple exercise took us on. As people began reading our prepared stories, they started telling us stories from their own lives. These stories really grabbed us, and we began writing them down. It is often said that everyone has at least one good story in them, and we have found this to be true. We have found that people often have many good stories to share from their lives. It may be surprising to learn that people living with dementia can still remember and tell stories from their lives, but we have seen it happen over and over again.

Ginger's Story:

We are not talking here about autobiography nor or we discussing life histories, but rather we are talking about incidents, fleeting moments from a person's life that they share with us. For example, there was Ginger's story about how she met her husband. He was the brother of a girl that Ginger worked with in a factory during WWII. He was in the Navy and was home on leave when Ginger went to her friend's house for dinner. Ginger told us,

"We took one look at each other and it 'bif, bam boom!'"

They were married before his leave was over and he had to go back to the Navy and to the war. He survived the war and they were married until his death, some forty years later. This was just a brief moment in Ginger's long life, but of course, a seminal one for her and for her husband.

When we met Ginger, she spent most of her day sleeping in her wheel chair. She was often awake at night, and this schedule made it difficult for us and for the staff to engage with her. Ginger told us this story during one of her rare waking moments in the day. As we talked with her about her memories of the war, she revealed to us that she worked nights in the factory. Perhaps this could explain her sleeping patterns now, even all these years later? We asked Ginger if she would like to film her story about how she met her husband. She agreed and we made a very short film of Ginger telling us this story. Then, as we always do, we showed Ginger her movie.

At first, we were alarmed because when Ginger saw herself on the television screen, she asked us,

"Who is that old woman? How does she know all that stuff about my life?"

Ginger began to grow agitated and we thought that perhaps this was a mistake. But then, as she began to listen to the old *woman talking on the TV, Ginger became engrossed in the story. She began to agree with the old woman, and shake her head yes, that was right. She laughed out loud when the old woman on the TV said that it was 'bif, bam boom,' when Ginger met her husband.*

She clapped heartily when the film ended and was very much awake when she went to lunch that day. We were not sure if Ginger understood that the woman talking on TV was actually her, but then we overheard her talking to her lunch companions and saying,

"You are not going to believe this, but I was on TV today. I had my own show on TV!"

When we realized that some people who have dementia can still tell stories from their lives, we began documenting these stories in print and on film. We learned that it was very important to give people something to hold in their hands in order to prime the pump of memory. For Ginger, we happened to be visiting on Veteran's Day and we just happened to give her a little flag that had the Navy insignia on it. She recognized the flag and that was the prompt that opened the gates to her story of how she met her husband. This was just a happy coincidence for us. Later, we would deliberately bring in meaningful objects or photographs from people's lives to help give them some context for sharing stories from their lives.

We talk to family members, staff, and friends to find salient information about the people with whom we are working. Using this information, we find the keys to help unlock treasured memories.

James's Story:

We met James in a memory enhancement center. James had lived all of his life in a tiny, rural community. He was a very bright student and had been offered a scholarship to go to college, but he declined. James told us,

"I was too embarrassed to ask my dad and granddad if I could leave the farm. I knew they couldn't afford to pay someone to take my place."

So, James stayed working the tenant farm with his dad and granddad. Being such a bright person, though, James worked out a formula so that he would be able to buy himself his own bit of land. His granddad and his father both thought he was crazy to be trying to buy a farm in the middle of the depression. James was not deterred; he believed in his dream and he believed in his formula. James's formula was simple but effective. He learned to live on the money he made from selling milk and eggs; all of the money he made from selling his hogs, he saved toward the purchase of a farm. In a couple of years he had saved enough for a down payment on an eighty acre farm. In six years, using his formula, James had paid off his farm free and clear. He was modestly proud of this accomplishment and shared his formula for success with a sheepish grin.

When we first met James, we learned from the staff that he had been a well respected farmer in the area for years. We saw an aerial photograph of his farm that was framed and hanging in his room. With James's permission, we took the photograph off of the wall, and gave it to him to hold.

Looking at the photograph of the farm, James began to describe the out buildings, the crops, the animals and then he launched in to the wonderful story that he told us about buying his own farm during the depression. We printed this story up in a large font, with photos of farm life, and have shared James's story with people all over the United States.

We have shared James's story with people who are living with dementia, we have shared his story with family caregivers and professional caregivers and medical staff. We have told his story on the radio and at national conferences. It is a simple story, but it speaks to the grit, the determination, the hard work of this generation. It also speaks to the fear that some people felt during this tough economic time in our history. This story has resonance for older people who lived through the great depression as well as younger people who are now living through our own difficult economic times.

Rebecca's Story:

Another person who gave us a different version of life during the Great Depression was Rebecca. Rebecca lived in a sod house on the prairie when she was a young girl. When she was ten years old, her family moved to Chicago where she lived the rest of her life. When we met Rebecca, she was 95 years old and living in a long term care center. Rebecca was a great story teller and had collected stories throughout her long life. She was also a poet and a musician. We knew Rebecca for two years, and visited her weekly during that time. She told us wonderful stories, but never remembered our names, nor was she quite sure who we were. Rebecca did know that we enjoyed hearing her stories and so she was always happy to spend time with us. We recorded several of Rebecca's stories on film and in print. As with James, Rebecca's stories and films have traveled many miles since she first shared them with us. They delight audiences of all ages. Here is one of our favorite Rebecca stories:

THE BEST GIFT

The calendar said it was spring, but winter wasn't quite finished with us yet. This particular Saturday started with a cold rain and as the temperature continued to drop, the rain turned to sleet. The sidewalks were soon covered with ice. As I climbed the steps to the El train downtown after work, a flower vendor's colorful display caught my eye. It seemed so out of place to see fresh roses in that miserably cold corner.

They weren't long stemmed, but they were roses. Suddenly I felt a tremendous urge to buy a dozen and bring them to my friend, Mae. Mae was a soloist in our choir. I was her accompanist, and I admired her tremendously. This was during the depression, so even twenty- five cents was big money for me. The vendor gave me extra wax paper to protect the roses, and I headed for home.

My mom was appalled when I told her of my planned errand as I gulped down a little of her good dinner. Her words,

"In this weather?" showed her concern.

After another two blocks of slipping and sliding, a short ride on the Western Avenue streetcar and longer ride on the Milwaukee Avenue streetcar, plus three more blocks of walking, I reached her address- but no Mae! Her grimly angry mother-in-law told me,

"They've moved out!" After considerable pleading, she gave me their new address.

Another three block hike brought me back to Milwaukee Avenue and the factory type building indicated. No front entrance, no side entrance. After picking my way through mud and debris, I found a rickety door at the back of the building. Inside was a long, dark stairway. With my heart in my throat, I inched my way up the stairs and

knocked at the door. The door opened and Mae's husband stood in the doorway with their toddler in his arms. His inability to find employment had led to the quarrel with his parents and their asking him to move. He told me Mae was walking to her mother's home to ask for money for bread and milk for the baby.

By now, I was feeling that the roses were totally inappropriate, but her husband's eyes were glistening as he put them in a tall water glass. His voice wasn't quite steady as he told me,

"When Mae left to go to her mother's she said, 'I don't think there is one person in this whole world who cares whether we live or die!'"

They both told me afterward of the healing tears that flowed when Mae returned home to find roses waiting for her. Through the years she has often mentioned that little bunch of roses as the best gift she had ever received!

– The End

When we share Rebecca's story with various groups, we always ask this question: What color were the roses? Nine out of ten people say that the roses were red. Sadly, we never asked Rebecca that question, so the color of the roses will forever be a mystery. Rebecca's story of this gift of compassion and love during very tough times, gives us an intimate look into the Great Depression. We learn about the courage and toughness of a young girl as she set out on her mission to bring flowers to her friend. We also ask groups who read this story,

"Would you have had the courage to walk up those dark, rickety stairs on a cold, sleeting, wet night?"

This story and these questions create deep and thought provoking discussions. James, the farmer, and Rebecca, the pianist, were seemingly ordinary people living ordinary lives, but their stories are filled with the bravery and determination of a generation that lived through economic hard times and a world war. These stories resonate through generations to touch everyone who hears them.

Paul's Story:

Finally, there was the love story that was told to us by a highly regarded scientist. He had taught in a major university and conducted important research that had an impact on world wide crop development. Knowing his life work, we brought in small galvanized buckets of different types of grains for him to put his hands into, to feel the grain again, to prime his memory of the years that he researched and worked with arable crops.

As often happens to us in this work, Paul completely surprised us by his response to this grain exercise. He happily plunged his hands into the buckets, letting the showers of grain slide through his fingers. His eyes took on a dreamy look as the grain fell from his fingers back into the bucket. Then, to our amazement, Paul, the scientist, began to tell us about his one great love, the girl who got away, the reason he never married.

Paul met her when he was working for the government in Washington D.C. When he began to describe Sherry, his whole physical being changed. His face turned bright pink, his eyes brightened and his breathing came in rapid breaths, as though he had been running. He never told us why they did not make a match of it, he only told us of his great love for her and of her personal loveliness.

We thought that by bringing in buckets of grain, Paul would tell us a story about his work in agricultural research, but instead we learned of his great love, Sherry. He said her name over and over again, with a dreamy smile on his face. It was a wonderful experience to see this great man of science talk about his one and only love, Sherry, the girl who got away.

GUIDEPOST:

People living with dementia have so much to teach us, so much to share with us of wisdom and joy and heartache and fortitude.

There have been books and articles written about "the storied memory." Stories are how we frame the scenes from our lives; it is how we remember our lives. People living with dementia obviously cannot remember their lives chapter and verse; they may be confused as to what era they are presently living in, or they may not remember events in the correct sequence, but there are scenes, moments from their lives that can be brought back to life. We know that the people telling us these amazing stories may not remember us or the stories they have told us; but we will never forget them or their stories. These stories bolster our belief that people who are living with dementia have so much to teach us, so much to share with us of wisdom and joy and heartache and fortitude. When we help people who are living with dementia bring their stories back to life, we give them the opportunity to be generative again, to give these stories from their lives back to their immediate communities, to their families and to the larger world.

CHAPTER SEVEN:

Lady Madonna

Maria's Story:

One of the life stories that had a profound influence on our work is the story of Dr. Maria Montessori, the first woman in Italy to become a physician. After much struggle and many hardships, Montessori was granted her medical degree and was immediately assigned to a position in an insane asylum in Rome. Living in this asylum were children of the inmates and children who were deemed to be "defective." These children were considered by most doctors and teachers of the time to be unteachable, unreachable.

Dr. Montessori's job was to care for the physical needs of these children, but she quickly realized that her young patients needed much more than medical care. Montessori noticed that the children would pick up scraps of food from the floor and roll it around in their hands. They had no other source of stimulation; they rarely, if ever, were allowed to go outside, and there were no opportunities for learning. Through trial and error and observation, Dr. Montessori began to develop hands-on learning tools. She discovered that these children could be reached by engaging their hands and their senses. After several years of working with these deprived and "defective" children, Dr. Montessori had her patients formally tested. Much to everyone's amazement, the children living in the asylum in Rome tested as well or better than school children in Rome!

Maria Montessori began to develop a pedagogy based on all she had discovered in her work in the asylum. The Italian government asked her to create a school for the very poor children living in the infamous San Lorenzo slums of Rome. Dr. Montessori quickly discovered that the children living in these desperate slums first needed to learn how to care for themselves and their environment. She created exercises for the children to practice activities of daily living so that they could live healthy, independent lives. After the children in the San Lorenzo slums learned how to take care of themselves and their environment, Dr. Montessori began to give them the learning tools that she had created for the children in the asylum. These learning tools were based on learning through doing, and by allowing the children as much time as they needed to repeat the learning experience. This school in the slums of Rome was the first of thousands of her Casa Dei Bambini (Children's Houses). Today, Montessori schools are found all over the world.

Hopefully, Dr. Montessori's story is interesting to you but what on earth does this story have to do with our work with people who are living with dementia? Just like the children that Dr. Montessori met in the asylum in Rome, people living with memory loss are often considered by the larger world to be "unreachable." But they are not, in fact, unreachable. There are several reasons that support our use of the Montessori Method to reach people living with dementia. First of all, this method is strength based. Dr. Montessori believed that it is essential to find the strengths, interests, and passions of people. It is easy to find all of the things that are deficits in people who have dementia, but there can still be remaining strengths and spared abilities. If we base our approach on using people's remaining interests and abilities, we have a much greater chance for success in reaching them and making meaningful connections.

GUIDEPOST:

The Montessori Method is based on finding people's remaining strengths and their spared abilities.

The second reason that we use the Montessori Method in our dementia work is that this method is based on the procedural learning system. As explained in Chapter Three, the procedural memory system tends to be less affected by dementia. We use many of the tools that Dr. Montessori developed because they are meaningful and attractive to all people, whether the person using the learning tool is 3 or 83. For example, we have had great success with Dr. Montessori's *Knobbed Cylinders* exercise. (*see* **figure 7**) This is a long block of wood with ten cylinders resting in ten holes. The cylinders are different shapes and sizes, and there is a self-correcting part to the exercise, as each cylinder will only fit in one hole. As in all of the Montessori tools, there is an element of natural beauty to this work that draws people to it.

We have seen people with dementia do this exercise and struggle to find the right cylinders. We can modify the exercise so that people will have success with it. For example, we will take out only three of the cylinders to simplify the exercise. So, only three holes need to be filled instead of ten. Or, if necessary, we will take out only one cylinder. We have seen many people with dementia gradually have more and more success with these types of exercises. Even though they will not remember having done the knobbed cylinders before, once the cylinder is in their hands, their muscle memory (procedural memory) kicks in and they can begin to build on what they learned about this work. Over time, we have observed people with dementia actually learning to do Montessori exercises because they were given the opportunity to learn at their own pace, in their own time, without being pressured or judged. They were able to use their muscle memory, the procedural memory system that is less affected by dementia, and so they were able to experience once again the good feeling that comes with success.

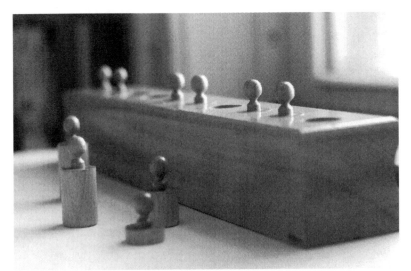

figure 7 - Knobbed cylinders exercise.

Everyone likes to feel that they can accomplish the task at hand, so we accommodate that basic need. We have discovered that if we give a person with memory loss the opportunity to work with Montessori materials repetitively, they can improve in their ability to do this work! They actually learn how to do the work better, how to do it faster and with more ease. Why is this important for someone who is living with dementia? What possible difference could this make to the quality of their lives or the lives of people who care for them? What does success with some wooden cylinder block mean to someone who is living with this condition?

> # GUIDEPOST:
>
> The Montessori Method is based on the procedural memory system. What we discovered that was truly amazing is this: If we give a person with memory loss the opportunity to work with Montessori materials repetitively, they can improve in their ability to do this work.

As stated earlier, success matters to everyone. When we accomplish a task, we feel better about ourselves and more confident. If someone is living with a condition that is confusing, frustrating and even terrifying, giving them the opportunities to be successful, even in a very simple task, can help bring forth feelings of calmness and the feeling of having some measure of control in their lives. On a more basic level, being able to use the pincer movement, being able to practice hand/eye coordination, also increases the ability of a person to handle activities of daily living, like being able to zip a jacket, or use a fork or spoon. (*see figure 8*)

Maintaining these activities helps us maintain some independence, some sense of accomplishment, some sense of control over the chaos that dementia can create in a person's life.

GUIDEPOST:

When we accomplish a task, we feel better about ourselves, more confident.

Our third reason for using the Montessori Method is that this method has been researched and codified. We not only have the proof of our own success in using this method, we can also point to the research that proves this success. While our work is grounded in the Montessori Method, we also create our own exercises and our own materials.

To sum up, we use the Montessori philosophy as our foundation for interacting with people living with memory loss because this philosophy is based on finding and building on the strengths of each person. The Montessori philosophy also teaches us to work with the whole person and to pay attention to the intellectual, physical and spiritual components of each individual. Dr. Montessori believed devoutly that every person deserves to be treated with respect and compassion. She encouraged us to celebrate our individual gifts and to

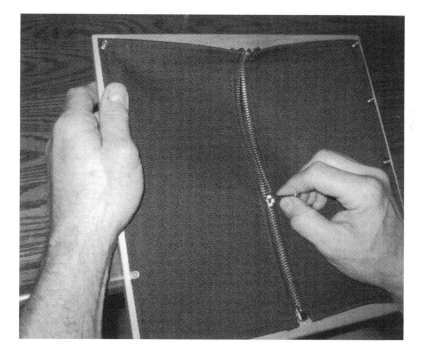

recognize each person's abilities. We use Montessori materials as prototypes to create new experiences for those living with dementia. Through the Montessori materials, we learn that every exercise we create should be beautiful, in good order, made with natural materials and based on the individual interests of the person.

> # GUIDEPOST:
>
> The Montessori Method has been researched and codified.

Some of our most astonishing experiences in using the Montessori Method for dementia care have happened

> # GUIDEPOST:
>
> It is a truly wondrous experience to see the power of the Montessori materials being shared by the very young and the very old.

when we created intergenerational programs. There is a kind of magic that happens when we bring young children and elders together. These two generations seem to understand each other. This is not to say that older people are childlike, but that both groups are innocent of hidden agendas, power plays and phony emotions. With both groups, elders and young children, what you see is pretty much what you get. They seem to understand and appreciate this lack of pretense and are amazingly comfortable with each other.

This may sound like we are painting with a large brush, but we have witnessed this phenomenon many, many times over the years in all sorts of situations. It is always the same; the young children and elders are drawn to each other.

We introduce Montessori materials and exercises into these intergenerational programs as a common tool that the older people and young children can work on together. Sometimes, the older person is the teacher and sometimes the child is the teacher. The roles go back and forth quite easily. Both groups understand that they are working on these projects together. They understand that they are there to support and help each other. It is a truly wondrous experience to see the power of the Montessori materials being shared by the very young and the very old.

Jake's Story:

Jake was a very violent person when his family brought him to the retirement community. He had been kicked out of four other facilities for his violent behavior. This particular home was known for its ability to work with people who had dementia and behavior problems. When we met Jake, he had already thrown four different televisions through four different windows. Jake was a tall, lanky man with the face of an aging film star, and a rare, but engaging crooked smile. His children stated that this rage and violence was completely out of character for their dad. He had been an affable, social person throughout his life. Jake had been an outdoors kind of man and hated being confined indoors. He and his wife owned a small landholding and Jake had enjoyed taking care of the lawn and garden at his home.

Because Jake was in good shape physically, the doctor gave him permission to be in charge of mowing the small lawn at the retirement community. Jake used an old fashioned, manual grass cutter and was very calm and rational while working out of doors in the yard and garden. He grew tomatoes, okra and onions for the kitchen at the home and took great pride in his crops. In the winter, Jake was in charge of feeding the birds and sweeping the paths. This outdoor work helped Jake calm down and gradually, over many months, he slowly became again the nice guy that his family remembered.

Jake really came into his own, though, when he was part of the group of elders who worked with the young children from the facility's daycare center. Once a week, the children, aged three to five, would come to visit a group of elders in Jake's home. The staff used Montessori materials and exercises for the group in their weekly meetings. One group would work on flower arranging, another group might work on a reading exercise, or painting together. Jake was particularly fond of the knobbed cylinder exercise. He appreciated the beauty of the wood and the precision with which the materials had been made. Jake would often pick up one of the cylinders and remark about how well made it was. When Jake first began working with the children on the knobbed cylinders, they were his teachers. He really struggled trying to figure out which cylinder belonged in which hole. The children were wonderfully patient with him, presenting the exercise to him the same way their teachers had shown it to them. He was allowed to experiment while they watched patiently. They only gave him help when he began to grow frustrated. As time went on, Jake was able to do this work faster and with more confidence. Even though he never remembered having done the work the week before, once the cylinders were placed in front of him, he picked them up with confidence and gradually he could do the work successfully without help from the children. We have a film of Jake successfully completing this work, the children clapping for him, and then he grins that charming, lop sided grin, and waggles his baseball cap before joining in the applause and clapping for himself. It is a moment that will live forever in our memories.

Veronica's Story:

We have seen the magic of Montessori and two different generations many times. Another time that stands out for us was one summer day with Veronica. Veronica was a gentle woman who could no longer speak. Her doctors, the staff and her family believed that dementia had caused her to completely lose her ability to use language. She smiled often and would sometimes watch our work with interest. She was still able to join in singing with the choir that had been formed in the retirement home, but she had not said a word in months.

This particular afternoon, Veronica sat with a group of little boys, watching while they worked on some geometric puzzles. When they were able to complete the puzzles successfully, Veronica would smile broadly and hit the table beside them in a movement of encouragement.

We knew that Veronica loved flowers and so we brought over the flower arranging exercise for this group. Veronica began helping the boys trim the flower stems and place the flowers in the vases. Then, to our utter amazement, Veronica began asking the boys to hand her things. She would ask for a vase or the scissors, just as though she had been speaking on a regular basis all along! We collectively held our breath while Veronica continued to work with the boys, talking to them about the flowers and the work that they were doing.

When the children left, we filmed Veronica as she talked to us about the children. She had some very profound things to say about children. She talked to us about her belief that children were good, that it was the things that happened to them later on in life that turned some of them bad. Veronica was thoughtful and eloquent on this subject.

As the following days went by, Veronica returned to her silence. She was pleasant, she smiled and sometimes joined in activities, but she did not speak. When the children returned for their next visit, Veronica would again speak to them; when they left, she would lapse into her silent self. This was the pattern that would continue for Veronica. No one could explain how or why it happened. It was as though the children unlocked something inside of Veronica. Whatever the reason, it was a little miracle to watch Veronica chatting with *the children during each of their visits. This is one of many small miracles we have observed in our work with Montessori and intergenerational programs.*

CHAPTER EIGHT:

With a Little Help from My Friends

BETTY WAS FILLING the watercolor paper with multi-colored dots. Dots of blue and green and yellow and pink were raining down everywhere on the paper. Suddenly, Betty stopped and looked questioningly at the aide sitting next to her.

"Is this alright? I am doing this right?" Betty asked about her painting project.

The aide smiled and shook her head.

"Don't worry, Betty. There is no right or wrong way to do a painting. Anyway, you are a regular Mozart!"

The resident aide had just completed a training session with us, and had received loudly and clearly our message that there is no right or wrong way to create a work of

GUIDEPOST:

<u>The Rule of Three:</u>

Is it true?

Is it necessary?

Is it kind?

art. This aide was a little confused about the role that Mozart had played in history, but the warmth of her smile and the encouragement in her voice gave Betty the incentive to continue working on her painting. We did not correct the aide and tell her that Mozart was a famous composer, not an artist; that would have been going against one of our own core beliefs. We look for the meaning behind the words, and it was very clear that day that the resident aide meant to encourage Betty, not give her a lesson in Western culture. It is so easy to jump in and correct anyone, someone living with dementia, or someone trying to help them. Before we get busy inserting ourselves into situations, we should remember the Rule of Three. This Rule of Three is at the heart of our philosophy of caregiving. We try to always stop and ask ourselves these questions before we jump in.

When we apply the Rule of Three before we act, we give ourselves that small moment to think and reflect before interjecting ourselves into a situation. Taking the time to reflect, to run through a brief mental review before we leap into action is helpful in caregiving.

Taking that brief moment before we act is very important when we are trying to help a person who is dealing with the phenomenon understood as failure to initiate; feeling confused about what steps must be taken to begin an activity. Tasks that seem simple, like remembering which clothes to put on first when getting dressed, or remembering what to do first when making coffee or loading a washing machine, can become confusing to people living with dementia. This is also very common, as most people living with dementia experience failure to initiate. In fact, the first signs of confusion are usually seen in a person's difficulty remembering how to begin routine tasks. We have learned to help people through this problem by doing the work with them. The key here is that we do the work with them, not for them.

GUIDEPOST:

We do the work with them, not for them.

For example, we may set up a painting exercise by attaching medium-sized paper to a table easel or board. [Paper that is too large may seem intimidating.] We set out no more than three dishes with paint in them and a couple of brushes and water. For some people with dementia, all of this painting paraphernalia is overwhelming, especially if they have never painted in their lives. We once had an elderly farmer tell us,

"I spent my whole life milking dairy cows. I can milk a cow for you, but I don't think I can paint you a picture." He did, in fact, paint a wonderful picture and went on to paint many times and truly enjoy it.

When a project seems intimidating, we have several techniques to help the person with dementia figure out how to approach the activity. As stated above, we can begin to do the work with them. We pick up a paint brush and start to paint and ask them to join us. Sometimes, just watching someone else do the work helps the person with dementia figure out how to begin the process. When introducing painting to someone living with dementia, we might begin by just asking them to dip the brush in paint; that is all we would accomplish that day. After the person has done this many times over the course of days or weeks, then we might ask them to just dab some color on the paper. It sometimes takes a tremendous effort on the part of the person with dementia to just make the brush touch the paper. We have often sat for ten minutes or more while the person tries to get the brush tip on the paper. If this experience sounds like it would be a frustrating experience for both them and us, we have to tell you that it is not frustrating, it is an amazing experience! There is, sometimes, that desire to just help them move the brush closer to the paper, but that would be defeating the entire goal of the exercise (which to is to do the work *with* but not *for* the person.) So, we sit and wait. We may pick up a brush and just touch the paper with a dot of paint ourselves. Sometimes, this helps to encourage the person who is struggling; sometimes we just have to wait. When the person living with dementia does finally touch the paper with the paint brush, it is often as though something inside of them has been unlocked. Not always, but often, we have witnessed people become completely absorbed in their painting. They may do abstract swirls or dots, or they may try their hand at some representative painting. (Houses are very common.)

Whatever art work they produce, it is wonderful to see how relaxed and how absorbed they are in the work itself. We are a creative species. Maybe we haven't painted anything since elementary school, but that impulse to create lives with us always, whether we nourish it or not. Even if we don't always recognize it in ourselves, we are all creative! Our creativity can take on many forms, of course. It can be painting, or writing poetry, or telling jokes, or sewing, cooking, gardening, problem solving, playing music or singing. Every time we turn our hand or our thoughts or our spirit to the act of creation, we are making something out of nothing. We fill the blank paper, we fill empty stomachs, we fill the barren plot, we fill lonely hearts, and we fill the lost soul. People living with dementia still have the need to create. It is our job to help them find opportunities where they can be successful in their creativity. To accomplish this, we need to understand the interests and passions of the people we care for. We also need to organize the creative experience so that it is accessible for the person with dementia. We can create the small steps necessary to help each person know once again the joy of creating something that can be shared and enjoyed by others.

GUIDEPOST:

We are all creative!

We use this technique of breaking activities down into very small steps in all of the work we introduce to people living with dementia. For example, if someone is joining a bread baking exercise, they may feel overwhelmed by all of the ingredients and the number of steps involved in the bread making process. We can give them one or two things to do (sifting flour or measuring the salt). Breaking down activities into smaller steps can be used throughout the course of the day. We can help someone dress appropriately by laying out the clothes in the order they should be put on. In doing this, we also help the person dress appropriately for the weather or the upcoming daily routine. We should discuss with the person what they want to wear that day, or give them choices between two things they might like to wear.

Again, we are not doing the work for them, but we are trying to give them the support they need to be successful in the activity, whether it is an activity of daily living, or some act of creativity. Dr. Montessori famously wrote,

"Every unnecessary aid is a hindrance."

This philosophy is true when teaching anyone, at any age or ability level. We are at our most helpful when we learn when and how to intervene. When and how depends on the individual we are helping and their own, particular set of circumstances.

Learning how to break down large projects into small steps is a lesson that is helpful to everyone, not just people living with dementia. We were once asked by a friend to help her clean up her father's house. Her dad was in the hospital recovering from a heart attack. This wasn't an ordinary clean up job. Our friend's father not only had a house crammed with years of clutter, there were also dirty dishes piled all over the kitchen, on the back porch, even the back steps! The place was a huge, gigantic mess. We stood gob-smacked, wondering where in the world we could begin.

We remembered all of the training classes we had given on caregiving and our mantra of "Break it down, break it down!" So, we took a deep breath and began the cleaning process by tackling one small square of space in the kitchen. Once that small space was clean, we moved onto another small space. After four days of back breaking work, we had cleaned the entire downstairs. There was still the upstairs to tackle, but we knew that we could succeed if we just broke the job down into small steps.

Here is what we did not understand at this time: We should not have cleaned up this person's house. We were doing the work for them, not with them, and of course, our friend's father was not happy with us or with the work we had done. We had forgotten one of the most important rules of "A Little Help from Our Friends": The help we give has to be wanted; the help we give needs to be a shared experience. Help is something that is done WITH, not done TO.

Our friend should have asked her father's permission before we began.

However, this exercise in breaking down the massive undertaking into a series of smaller, more manageable steps proved incredibly helpful and kept us from feeling overwhelmed by the big picture. This advice works wonders for people living with dementia as they face each new task. Remembering to tackle each caregiving job by breaking it down into small steps is also very helpful to caregivers. We have used this technique in so many moments in our lives, from new work projects to career changes to facing serious illness. Just take one small step at a time. Encourage the people living with dementia to join you in taking each small step.

> # GUIDEPOST:
>
> "Every unnecessary aid is a hindrance"
> – Dr. Maria Montessori

ACTIVITY:
FLOWER ARRANGING

The Montessori Method encourages the use of real world, natural and beautiful materials. Keeping real flowers on dining tables or in common areas of the environment can lift the spirits and cheer people, even on the gloomiest days. Bringing nature into the environment can also be very calming. Giving people with dementia the opportunity to be creative and to contribute to their community is very important for maintaining existing skills and for encouraging self-esteem. Pouring water into vases, cutting stems and arranging flowers all call on small motor movements, skills that are essential for independence and range of motion. *(see **figure 9**)* Touching the real flowers, smelling them and looking at the flowers call on the use of several senses, which is very helpful when engaging persons who have dementia. Making judgments of how much to trim off the stems, and which flowers go where bring into use the cognitive and artistic parts of the brain.

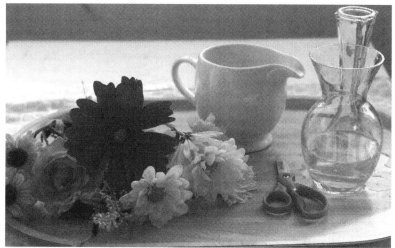

figure 9 - Items needed for flower arranging exercise.

MATERIALS NEEDED			
Real Flowers (thorns removed)	Vases	Pitcher	Funnel
Basket	Safety Scissors	Cloths	Cutting board
If possible, basket, cloths, scissors and funnel should be the same color or in the same color family.			

PURPOSE
To give participants the opportunity to be creative.
To give participants the opportunity to add beauty to their environment and their community.
Range of motion in placing flowers in vases.
Small motor control in using scissors and pouring water into vases.
Cognitive stimulation in measuring size of flowers and size of vases.

PROCEDURE
Invite participants to cut flowers to match vases, removing extra leaves and stems.
Invite participants to pour water into vases, using funnel if necessary
Allow participants to arrange flowers in vases any way they wish
Place flower arrangements on dining room tables or in common area
With participants, throw away stems and leaves
Help participants mop up any spills with cloths
Return basket to shelf

If a person cannot do all of the steps to the flower arranging exercise, just give them one or two simple things to do: Have them pour the water in the vases, or have them hand the flowers to the person arranging the flowers in the vases. We don't say that a person cannot be successful in any given exercise; we find a way to help them be successful by tailoring the work to each person's ability.

Giving people the opportunity to be successful often leads to their becoming more confident, more calm, more engaged in the present moment. Having this kind of engagement gives people with dementia the opportunity to open up about their own lives. We have learned so many important life lessons in these moments of engagement. When we talk of a little help from our friends, we mean that the pendulum swings both ways. As caregivers, we always think that we are there to help; it is our job, our calling, our burden, our gift. However we characterize it, caregivers, whether family, friends, or professional know that their work is to help others. Here is the interesting part, the part that took us by surprise and continues to take us by surprise. This helping thing does not go in only one direction. Caregivers are often the recipient of great gifts of wisdom, humor, courage and patience. We were really not prepared at all for the many and varied gifts that people living with dementia would give to us, the real help they would give to us in our lives.

The thing is, we have to be ready to receive these gifts from the people for whom we are caring. It is common in our culture to portray elders as cranky, difficult, petulant, and selfish. There are, no doubt, elders with these negative attributes, just as there are younger people who are difficult, demanding, greedy, pessimistic. All of us, no matter what our age, have unpleasant and difficult parts of our personality; this is not unique to elders. What is special about many elders is that they have learned through their long lives to see and understand patterns in life, the warp and woof of our behavior.

Many elders that we have met in this work help us see the funny side to life.

People often ask us how we can bear to work with people living with dementia. They tell us how depressing and sad the work must be, how dismal, how draining. In the past, we tried to explain to these people who felt so sorry for us, that they were wrong, that there is a lot of laughter and good times in our work. However, we have since learned not to argue with people who insist that our work is sheer drudgery. They do not want to believe that elders, especially those living with dementia, could ever be any fun. They simply will not accept that there is a lot of joy and sustained, outright laughter with the people we meet in this work. This ability to be able to laugh at some of the rotten things that life throws at us has been a huge help in our own lives. We try and give a little help to our friends, and they reward us with large gifts of laughter.

The wisdom thing is something, too. Other cultures seem to understand and appreciate the wisdom of their elders much more than we in Western cultures do. Dr. Bill Thomas, the well-known geriatrician, writer and developer of the Eden Alternative and the Greenhouse Project, says that we give the wrong tests to our elders. In our culture, we tend to judge elders on tests that are more appropriate for someone who is 35 years old, not 85 years old. We judge our elders negatively because they cannot move or think as quickly or as fluidly as someone in their 30s. Elders fail all of the tests that judge a person on strength, endurance and speed. But, Dr. Thomas points out that spiritually and emotionally elders will kick your butt! Elders may have lost or be losing their visual acuity, but their spiritual acuity is razor sharp. They may not be able to run fast, or jump high anymore, but they can make tremendous imaginative leaps with us, if we ask them to. Their hearing may be going but their ability to really listen and to understand life experiences is strong and deep.

Melba's Story:

Melba had been raised in the mountains of Appalachia, the oldest girl in a family of twenty children. Melba could recall sleeping head to toe with several siblings in one bed. She also remembered how her mother would never eat with the family, but survived on scraps left after her brood had finished eating. When she was a teenager, Melba would sit with her mother while the rest of the family ate. She told us that she felt it was her honor to sit with her mother, quietly watching while the rest of the family ate their dinner. Melba was not well educated and had worked hard, physical jobs her entire life. When she was a girl and young woman, she spent her days picking cotton and doing other field work. Melba took great pride in the fact that while other field hands peed on their sacks of cotton to make it heavier at the weigh- in, she refused to resort to this sort of practice. She felt it was cheating and it was not lady like.

When Melba married and moved away from her beloved mountains, she worked other back breaking jobs. One of these jobs was in a steel foundry. She had been hired to haul oily sand in a wheel barrow from one end of the dark, overheated foundry to another part of the steel mill. It was like working in hell, Melba told us. However, her husband had left her for another woman and she had three children to raise, so she took whatever work she could find. The foundry was one of the few places hiring. Melba took this back breaking, soul destroying work in order to provide for her family.

Melba was a person who had known deprivation, hard work and heartache most of her life. Now, she was old, her body tired and used up and she was living with Alzheimer's. There didn't seem much to celebrate in Melba's life, but whenever we worked with her, she was unfailingly cheerful, always so delighted to work with us and ever willing to try new things. Melba had a saying that she never failed to express when we met with her. Her bottom lip would tremble, and her eyes would fill with tears and Melba would say to us,

"We have so much to be thankful for in this life, and we don't thank God enough, do we? There is always something to be thankful for."

Melba told us this every single time we met with her. This woman, who had known poverty, struggle and heartache her entire life, believed that there was so much in life for which we should be grateful. We made Melba a little sign that she hung over her bed. The sign read,

"There is always, always something to be grateful for!" Whenever we start to feel put upon or churlish, we remember Melba, and we remember to take a moment to be grateful.

We give a little help to the friends we have met in this dementia work and they have given to us in return so much more than we could have ever expected. What is always thrilling for us is that so many people living with dementia can still be creative, and can sometimes be the one who touches our hearts and fills up our souls. Caregiving can be a reciprocal experience, if we allow those we care for to give a little help to us, their caregivers and their friends.

Jo's Story:

Jo is one of the people we met who taught us important lessons about the power of creativity and the unflagging strength of the human spirit. Jo is in her eighties and trying to cope with the twin blows of living with Parkinson's and Alzheimer's. We watch as she applies paint to paper. Because of the Parkinson's disease, Jo's hand shakes so badly that she must cup her left hand around her right arm in order to steady her brush. While she paints, Jo tells us that artists and writers and gardeners should remember that nothing in nature is perfect. She points out that even the most beautiful flower petals can look ragged and torn upon close inspection. We watch Jo continue to work on her portrait of a single, red rose. She creates shadows and depths in different shades of red, while the leaves of the flower trail away from the shimmering rose, curling and turning with patches of brown and pink and shadings of green. Jo layers paint, rubbing the excess off with her thumb, while the rose and its leaves and stem become luminous under her touch. We promise Jo that we will have this glorious rose framed, and that we will bring it back when we come to visit her again in the Memory Enhancement Center where she now lives.

When we meet Jo again, we hand her the painting, matted and framed, the rose looking even more alive, more vibrant under the glass. Jo looks at us blankly, not remembering us, not remembering her painting. Jo shakes her head and tells us that this is not her work, she does not, cannot paint anymore. Then a sudden smile lights up her face and Jo tells us that she will hang the rose painting in her room; it might inspire her to try her hand at art again.

Relentlessly, Parkinson's and dementia are destroying Jo's mind and her body, but within this destruction there still lives the artist, the creator. Once again, we hand Jo a paintbrush. This time, an entire garden of flowers jumps to life under her shaking hand. Watching Jo's courageous brush strokes, the words of Ernest Hemingway come to mind:

"The world breaks everyone, and afterward many are strong at the broken places."

CHAPTER NINE:

Do You Want to Know a Secret?

SOME OF THE very best experiences we've had are when we incorporate music into our work. People who may never speak, or have trouble finding common words can still often sing and remember all of the words to favorite songs or hymns. The voices may not be as strong as they were years ago. There may be more quavering notes but the love of singing is still strong in so many of our elders. Their generation was one that sang a lot, whether in church or synagogue, in school chorus, or just singing together with friends on the street corner, this was a singing generation!

Anyone who has ever sung in a chorus understands the strong bonds and the joy that group singing can bring. Many elders have never forgotten this experience, nor have they forgotten the songs. These songs uplifted and unified this older generation in a way that nothing else really could. This music can still uplift and unify them today.

> # GUIDEPOST:
>
> People who may never speak, or have trouble finding common words, can still often sing, and remember all of the words to favorite songs or hymns.

When we play the word finding exercise, "Name This Tune" (see Chapter Five) people who play the game with us begin to sing the tunes spontaneously. Suddenly, there is a group sing along and the people in the group sometimes remember all of the verses in a song! These are people who may not remember the names of their family members. They may not be able to name simple objects like a table or a toothbrush, but they remember every word to their favorite song. Singing is a procedural memory exercise, so it is a spared ability. There is also just something in music that lights up the brain, something that calls forth memory. This is the secret that we happily share with you: music is a direct route to reach people living with dementia.

Music is a direct route to reach people living with dementia.

People who were able to play a musical instrument in their earlier lives can usually still play that instrument when they are living with dementia. (Again, procedural or muscle memory preserves this knowledge.) They may be rusty, they may have lost much of their proficiency with the instrument, but they can often still play something. Here is another important secret: If given the opportunity, people with dementia can practice on their instrument and they can get better! We know because we have seen it happen.

Dom's Story:

Dom had been a pianist and choral teacher all of his adult life. When we met him, he had been living with dementia for many years. Living in a locked dementia unit, Dom became withdrawn, belligerent and difficult to deal with. However, when he sat down at the piano in the gathering room of the long-term care home, he could play tunes from memory for hours! He was a wonderful musician who played with flourishes, panache and with great joy. His whole face would light up and he would become lost in the music. People would spontaneously gather around the piano and join in singing as Dom played.

There was just one little blip in this magical musical recital of Dom's. Somewhere in every song, he would insert a phrase or two of the tune, Listen to the Mockingbird and he would whistle along to the snatches of this song. Dom could be in the middle of a fabulous rendition of Unchained Melody, or building to the ending of My Country Tis of Thee and then, suddenly, up would pop Listen to the Mockingbird with Dom whistling away. The singers that usually joined Dom in his impromptu concerts were amazingly tolerant of this little musical quirk of his. They would either try to sing a couple of lines from Listen to the Mockingbird, or they would patiently wait for the whistling to die away and for Dom to return to the original song. He always would return to the song, and to our astonishment, he would pick up the tune right where he left off before it was interrupted by his signature tune and his whistling. Dom was a happy man when he sat down to play the piano. That was the only time we ever saw him be gregarious, relaxed and happy. Music was the one thing that seemed to reach him. Through the music, Dom gave himself and many others hours of unadulterated joy.

One of the most enjoyable times in our work is when we bring out drums for a drum circle. (*see* **figure 10**) We meet people who tell us they can't play drums because they don't have any rhythm. We tell them that if they have a heart beat, then they have rhythm in their bodies. We have used all sorts of drums for this work, including large gathering drums with mallets. These drums can be played by five or so people, all playing this one drum together. The remarkable secret about the gathering drum experience is that, after a short time, the group begins hitting the drum at the same time, using the same beat. They usually begin in a sort of chaos of sound, and

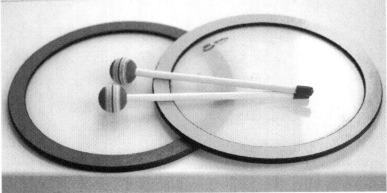

figure 10 - Frame drums exercise equipment.

then, gradually, they find a common beat and they all begin to hit the drum together. We were stunned the first time we saw this happen. People were actually listening to each other and then began playing the drum with each other. It is a wonderfully bonding experience.

GUIDEPOST:

If you have a heart beat, then you have rhythm.

We also use smaller drums, such as an African djembe drum. This drum stands up in front of an individual and can be played by striking it with a soft mallet. Djembes come in several different sizes and have different tones, so that a chorus of these drums can sound quite musical. We also use small, thin, light framed drums. These can be from ten-inches across going down in circumference to five-inches across, each having a different tone. These can be played by hitting the drum head with the fingers. Whatever kind of drum we use, after a few moments of playing together, the drum circle becomes a cohesive unit, with the group starting and stopping together naturally. This natural cohesion, this ability to come together as a true musical group is a wonderful secret that we discovered much to our delight and amazement.

We see all sorts of drummers in our dementia drum circles. Some people use the drum as a means to release stress or anger. We see them beating the drum with all of their might, their mouths pursed tightly. After a time, these angry drummers begin to calm down, and to join in the rhythm of the circle. Their tight faces relax and the grimaces are replaced with smiles. We also see the shy drummers, people who tentatively and softly hit their drums. After a time, these shy drummers gradually lose their inhibitions and sometimes we see them wailing away on their drums, tapping their toes, completely absorbed in the rhythm surrounding them. There are many kinds of drummers in our drum circles, but, over time, everyone experiences their own happiness and a true bonding with others in the circle. Much of the fog and confusion of dementia starts to fall away in these drum circles and we see the joy of life come shining through the faces of the drummers.

There can be many types of drum circles, just as there are many types of drummers. Some drum circles are more formal. The leader may start the group out with simple rhythms, such as ma-ma, da-da, ma-ma, da-da. Gradually, the leader can add more simple rhythms, such as Mississippi-hot-dog, Mississippi-hot-dog. There are many simple rhythm patterns that can be used in this more formal approach to drum circles. A drum circle can consist of ten to twenty people, or it can simply be a caregiver and a person with dementia.

A less formal but equally productive type of drum circle would be one in which everyone sings and beats out time to the songs. This type of circle can be accompanied by someone on the piano or with a CD, or just with the voices of the people playing the drums. Any sort of upbeat songs will work in a sing along, drum along circle.

We frequently hold both types of drum circles, strictly rhythm pattern circles and the singing drum circles. Both are fun, both bring a group of people together, both are helpful for expressing emotions. For people who struggle with language, or who can no longer use language, drum circles are a wonderful way to express those emotions that they can no longer express through words.

Drumming gives people the chance to release pent up emotions, to share those feelings with a group, to find support from the circle and to join together to make a joyful noise.

CHAPTER TEN:

Let It Be

DOES THE IDEA of letting go, letting it be, mean that we are giving up, that this is all there is, that things will never be better, that we just have to sigh, shrug our shoulders, hang our head and simply say, 'Oh well, let it be'? Or could this concept of letting things be mean that we are not giving up, that to the contrary, we are feeling empowered? We can let go because we understand now that there is so much that we can do: we can change our attitude, we can change our language, we can look for and build on strengths, and we can celebrate small moments, tiny victories. We can work at living in just this moment, being thankful for the smile, the laugh, the squeeze of our hand, the shared time together.

We cannot change how other people feel about dementia. We cannot make them stop feeling afraid, or uncomfortable. It is hard enough to control these feelings in ourselves, we cannot hope to try and control these negative feelings in other people. Having read this book, you know now and understand that, while you cannot change the condition of dementia, you can change how you look at it and how you live with it.

How you live with dementia depends completely on your own attitude. We cannot change the condition itself, but we can change how we approach this enormous challenge in our lives. We are still in a relationship, even a partnership with the person we love who has dementia. However, we are the only partner in this relationship who can decide how to think, how to behave, what to believe, how to cope. The person living with dementia, obviously, is being propelled on a journey over which they have very little or no control. We still have control (even though it may often feel that we don't). We can still make attitude adjustments, course corrections, seek help and take time for ourselves. The person living with dementia has none of these choices available to them.

Caregiving is some of the most difficult and demanding work that we will ever do. It demands great patience and strength of character. It is a role for the courageous and the optimistic. You will probably have many moments of sorrow, even despair, but you will never, ever regret taking on this very difficult work. For the rest of your life, you will know that within you lives a hero. You will carry with you moments of tenderness and joy that can only come from the intimacy of caregiving. You will know that you faced the most daunting challenge of your life and met it head on. Even through your sadness and loneliness, you will gain comfort from the knowledge that you have done and are doing the very best that you could for the person you love. That is all any of us can do, just our very best.

You are learning in this caregiving journey the very important lesson that all of us must learn: You know that we can't control or even influence everything in our world. Those things we can't control or influence, we simply have to learn to LET IT BE!

> # GUIDEPOST:
>
> For the rest of your life, you will know that within you lives a hero!

While we are learning to let go, we are also trying to prepare for the final letting go; that moment when the person we care for will leave us forever. There is no real way to completely prepare for this eventuality. Even though we know that this is the final destination of You Say Good Bye and We Say Hello of dementia care, it is impossible to know how we will feel, how we will act when that final moment of letting go happens to us.

Even though we can't predict our emotional state at the moment of passing, we can make some practical plans that will help us when the moment comes. We would suggest making a list of people to call with their phone numbers listed. This list should be prioritized: Who is the person you most need to be with you in these final moments? This person or people should be at the top of your list. (We are not talking about emergency phone numbers, doctors' phone numbers, hospice and funeral home numbers. These are all important contacts that should also be with you.) What we are suggesting is creating in advance a list of people who will serve as your emotional support team. As you learned to do while you were a caregiver, don't be too shy or too proud to ask these people for their help. Give them specific things to do for you. Remember, these people are your support team. They want to help you. You have to let them.

GUIDEPOST:

Create a list of people who will serve as your emotional support team.

Grieving is a very personal experience; everyone deals with it in their own way. Some days, it is all a person can do to just get out of bed, brush their teeth and put one foot in front of the other. Some days, we can't even get out of bed at all. We do have one suggestion that has been very helpful to us in times of sorrow: Use the arts to express your grief: Writing, painting, playing music, singing, anything creative that can focus your mind and gives you an emotional outlet is so very helpful during the long months and even years of mourning.

Some people may feel they do not want to try the arts, that this approach would not be helpful to them. For those of us who feel this way, we would suggest going to see performances, listening to music, finding those books that speak to you. Bobby Kennedy said that reading poetry was a tremendous help to him as he mourned the tragic loss of his brother, President John Kennedy.

Grief is a long and winding road, with very few guide posts to show you the way to peace and understanding. While there will never be an end to grief, we can learn to live with it. Just as we learn to live with physical pain, we can find coping mechanisms and strategies to help us through this dark and lonely time. We have to remember, though, to give ourselves the time and the space we need to mourn. We have to be patient with ourselves.

The Victorians understood the importance of allowing people the time and the space to grieve properly. In those times, people wore black clothes or wore black arm bands for a year after the death of someone close to them. This type of dress was a sign to other people that this person was in mourning and needed to be treated with respect and understanding. Today, we have no outward sign to the world that we are in grief. Often, the best intentioned and well meaning people want us to "snap out it", "don't be depressed", and "just get over it…move on".

We need to acknowledge our feelings of sadness and loss. We need to let these feeling be, we need to feel them, and we need to walk through our days of mourning without guilt, without despair. Grieving is natural and so human. It is very painful and because of this pain, we often feel that emotion known as fight or flight; we want to deny or fight these waves of grief, or we just want to run away, to escape from these terrible feelings. But, we cannot run away from ourselves, or run away from our own sadness. We just have to walk through this experience, asking for specific help, leaning on our friends, family, and our faith. At some point, it will be the right time to try and move away from the all consuming grief, to let it go, let it be. We will never forget the person we cared for, but we can learn how to live again without them. They will go with us to this new life. The people we cared for and loved will be with us forever.

> # GUIDEPOST:
> We need to acknowledge our feelings of sadness and loss.

CONCLUSION:
And In the End

CARING FOR SOMEONE who is living with dementia may not seem world shattering to the caregivers who are preforming this exhausting and demanding task, but we should recognize the fact that every caring act helps to build a more caring world. Learning how to become a caregiver, how to truly care for another person's well being (emotionally, physically and spiritually) is a giant step forward in the evolution of the human soul.

GUIDEPOST:

Learning how to become a caregiver, how to truly care for another person's well being (emotionally, physically and spiritually) is a giant step forward in the evolution of the human soul.

Mahatma Gandhi once wrote that the only way to change the world is to do it one person at a time. He famously said,

"You must be the change you wish to see in the world."

It is our fervent hope that this book has given caregivers the necessary tools to help all of us become more successful, more understanding and more creative in this caregiving work. It was also our goal to create guideposts that can lead caregivers to a more positive approach to caregiving. Changing the way we think and speak about dementia can change how we see our role and how we perform that role. Seeing ourselves as heroes rather than victims or martyrs helps us understand the true nature of the work we are doing. When we understand the beauty and the dignity of caregiving, we can begin to see that caring for another person is a gift that has been given to us. Through the exhaustion and the frustration and the tears, we must still remember that the act of caring deeply for another person can bring forth the very best in us.

We should take a few moments each and every day and celebrate this gift of caring. If we look carefully, every day (even on the worst days) we can find some event that helps us celebrate caregiving. It may be something as small as a returned squeeze of the hand, or a fleeting smile or a flash of a shared memory. These tiny moments contain the joy and connection that make all of the difficult times worth it.

Without your sacrifice, your noble efforts, your great love, this world would be a much diminished place. Your caregiving work illuminates not only your own life and the life of the person for whom you care; your work lights the way for all who are trying to find their way through the world of dementia. We hope that you will share the tools and ideas in this book that you found to be helpful. All of the strategies and techniques written about in *You Say Good Bye and We Say Hello* are easily adaptable to many situations in life. Please use the lessons here to help you find your way through other difficulties you may face.

We look forward to hearing from you and discussing your ideas and your stories about the caregiving journey. Caregivers are, of course, a large and diverse group, but we all share the belief that we can learn to do our caring work better. One of the best ways to improve our own caregiving abilities is to learn from the successes and failures of others.

Finally, we want to tell you that we deeply respect and honor the work you do every day and every night: Stay strong, celebrate each tiny victory, laugh when you can and cry when you must. Remember how perfectly wonderful you are and how fortunate you are to be given the gift of caregiving.

And, in the end, the love you take is equal to the love you make.

TYPOGRAPHY FOR THIS BOOK

The main text (12pt), chapter titles (14pt-18pt) and headings (14pt) were set in Cardo, copyrighted and authored by David Perry (http://scholarsfonts.net/cardofnt.html) and licensed under the SIL Open Font License Version 1.1(http://www.fontsquirrel.com/license/Cardo) granting use of this font for personal and commercial use.

Guidepost headings (24pt), image descriptions (10pt), figures (12pt) and charts (10pt-12pt) are in Cabin, copyrighted by Pablo Impallari (http://www.impallari.com) and Igino Marini (http://www.ikern.com) and licensed under the SIL Open Font License Version 1.1 (http://www.fontsquirrel.com/license/cabin) for personal and commercial use.

Page numbers (13pt), footnotes (10pt), book title and author name (11pt) and text of Guideposts (14pt) was set in Quattrocento. This font is also copyrighted by Pablo Impallari and Igino Marini and licensed under the SIL Open Font License Version 1.1 (http://www.fontsquirrel.com/license/quattrocento-roman) for personal and commercial use.

A thank you to these type founders for their hard work in producing such impeccable fonts.

Made in the USA
Lexington, KY
25 July 2013